Acclaim for the writing of Niall McLaren, M.D.

"Dr. McLaren brilliantly wields the sword of philosophy to refute the modern theories of psychiatry with an analysis that is sharp and deadly. His own proposed novel theory could be the dawn of a new revolution in the medicine of mental illness."
—Andrew R. Kaufman, MD
Chief Resident of Emergency Psychiatry
Duke University Medical Center

"Not only does Dr. Niall McLaren point out the various shortcomings of the established views of psychology/psychiatry, and of some other scientific disciplines, but he also proposes the most cogent model of mind that does not violate fundamental scientific laws and is also compatible with the norms of common sense and logic. He has endangered the foundations of contemporary mainstream psychiatry while, at the same time, creating a rescue channel."
—Ernest Dempsey, editor of *Recovering the Self Journal*

"This book is a *tour de force*. It demonstrates a tremendous amount of erudition, intelligence and application in the writer. It advances an interesting and plausible mechanism for many forms of human distress. It is an important work that deserves to take its place among the classics in books about psychiatry."   —Robert Rich, PhD, AnxietyAndDepression-Help.com

"I found Niall McLaren's book to be an incredibly well-written and thought-provoking. It is not, by any means, easy reading. It is also not for someone who doesn't have some form of background in understanding the various psychological theories and mental health conditions. I think that this would make an excellent textbook for a graduate class that allows students to question the theories that we already have."
—Paige Lovitt for *Reader Views*

"It is impossible to do justice to this ambitious, erudite, and intrepid attempt to dictate to psychiatry a new, 'scientifically-correct' model theory. The author offers a devastating critique of the shortcomings and pretensions of psychiatry, not least its all-pervasive, jargon-camouflaged nescience."
—Sam Vaknin, PhD, author Malignant Self Love: Narcissism Revisited

"McLaren's book has been thirty years in the making and is obviously well researched and thought-out. The author makes very strong, intelligent arguments that, I believe, will have a large impact on the future of psychiatry. McLaren's book would make an excellent read for a psychiatry student or for those already in the field."
—Kam Aures for *Rebecca's Reads*

"This is an academic book about psychiatric methods. As a psychology graduate as well as a user of the various services, I find this a fascinating subject. It's not for a beginner, but for someone who has some experience of the mental health services, it's interesting and thought-provoking. We need to get over the stigma attached to mental health and see it on the same level as physical health issues. It's not a new theory, but more of an overview of what has gone before and where the future direction of psychiatry should lead."

—Josie Henley-Einion, author of *Silence*

"Among the theories McLaren shows as severely flawed are behaviorist models, psychoanalysis, and eclectic models of psychiatry. Most importantly, McLaren states that no real foundational theory exists for psychiatry. While definitions of mental disorder exist, no real definition of mental order or normality has been determined. Until it is determined what a normal mental state is, psychiatry cannot accurately determine what is a mental disorder.

McLaren's thesis is that 'human behavior is the outcome of a complex interaction between an emergent mind and the physical body.' While psychiatry has focused on depression as the most popular mental disorder, McLaren believes the focus should be on anxiety, which is the result of the 'fight or flight' instinct in most creatures; traumatic events that cause anxiety can lead to depression, so consequently anxiety deserves to be studied as a source of depression. McLaren emphasizes that the human mind does affect the human body, as in cases of mass hysteria, anxiety, and fear that create panic attacks.

Ultimately, McLaren says that any theory of the mind has to provide a rational explanation of mental disorder. He boldly speaks his mind throughout the book, backing up his points with multiple examples, and he is not afraid to cry "Humbug!" when necessary. McLaren has been practicing psychiatry since 1977 in Australia. His discussion of his own education and the shortcomings of the education system he went through as well as weaknesses in current psychiatric practices demonstrate that psychiatry has many more steps to take before it is a completely effective science. This work may well lead to a new understanding of mental illness in future years as younger psychiatrists read his book and follow his example in rejecting the ineffective theories he derides."

—Tyler R. Tichelaar, PhD

"This is a paradigm-challenging work, to say the very least, and McLaren's views require a person who has a vested interest in these subjects to confront their own resistance to challenge. It's worthwhile, because McLaren's book is affirmative concerning something which many people may have found lacking in modern psychology, and psychiatry: namely, a psyche.

With the technological revolutions occurring in the past century-and-a-half, it seems every scientist wanted to find a way to reduce the psyche to a physical property, or some combination of physical properties, or completely deny its existence (behaviorism). While this has certainly been in vogue, and has yielded many useful results in terms of understanding neurobiology and its connection to moods and perception, it has not been successful in penetrating an understanding of 'the Self', or the psyche. Some will say this is because the self/psyche doesn't exist, but is only a fiction that appears to the individual: still, this is just a reduction to absurdity- what is the person who perceives the self, but indeed the self?"

—Kevin Brady, *Clear Objectives*

HUMANIZING PSYCHIATRY: THE BIOCOGNITIVE MODEL

Niall McLaren, M.D.

*"Orthodoxy means not thinking—not needing to think.
Orthodoxy is unconsciousness."*
George Orwell, 1984

Library of Congress Cataloging-in-Publication Data

McLaren, Niall, 1947-
  Humanizing psychiatry : the biocognitive model / Niall McLaren.
      p. ; cm.
  Includes bibliographical references and index.
  ISBN-13: 978-1-61599-011-5 (trade paper : alk. paper)
  ISBN-10: 1-61599-011-9 (trade paper : alk. paper)
  ISBN-13: 978-1-61599-012-2 (hardcover : alk. paper)
  ISBN-10: 1-61599-012-7 (hardcover : alk. paper)
  1. Psychiatry--Philosophy. 2. Cognitive neuroscience. 3. Psychology,
Pathological. 4. Biological psychiatry. I. Title.
  [DNLM: 1. Psychiatry. 2. Models, Psychological. 3. Psychological Theory.
WM 100 M161h 2010]
  RC437.5.M44 2010
  616.89--dc22
                                    2009035242

Distributed by: Baker & Taylor, Ingram Book Group, Quality Books
Future Psychiatry Press is an imprint of
Loving Healing Press
5145 Pontiac Trail
Ann Arbor, MI 48105
USA

http://www.LovingHealing.com or
info@LovingHealing.com
Fax +1 734 663 6861

Future Psychiatry Press

For my wife and children.

Amici certi in re incerta

Contents

Table of Figures

Acknowledgement: I am grateful to Prof. Peter Somogyi, Dept of Pharmacology, University of Oxford, for permission to use Fig. 6-2.

Introduction

The whole point of a religious or political education is to do exactly as your teachers say. The whole point of a scientific education is to overthrow your teachers.

I-1. The Gathering Crisis in Psychiatry

Since my monograph, *Humanizing Madness: Psychiatry and the Cognitive Neurosciences*, was published in 2007, I have had the chance to meet people in the US, and keep regular email contact with people all over the world. Talking to medical students, psychiatry trainees and junior psychiatrists has convinced me that, unless there is a radical transformation, even a revolution in psychiatry, then the profession will more or less cease to exist within the next twenty years. Some people might retort: And not before time, but I will answer that later. Here, I will briefly outline why I have this gloomy view.

The first thing I noticed in the US was a widespread and profound disenchantment among trainees with what they are being taught. From what I can see (and I have nothing to do with psychiatric training in Australia), today's trainees don't have anywhere near the fun we had thirty years ago. There is no sense of excitement among our junior colleagues. Their academic courses consist of dredging through thousands of papers stuffed full of statistics, of pharmacology, of brain enzymes and fMRI scans and the like, but there is no humanity in it. These days, psychiatrists see patients for a short time, quickly announce a diagnosis according to the DSM-IV, write a prescription and hand the patient over to case managers. A month or more later, when the patient comes back for more prescriptions, he is just as likely to see another doctor. The intellectual and emotional satisfaction at being able to step inside patients' lives and see it from their point of view is simply not there. Psychiatry consists of drugs, one-size-fits-all programs, mission statements and endless forms to fill in.

The practice of psychiatry has been hammered into a bureaucratized and corporatized model of cut-price service delivery, where the demands of torts lawyers count for more than the needs of a person in pain. At an accelerating pace, psychiatry is being pared down. From my vantage point up here at the top of Australia, I see that hospital psychiatrists no longer take calls; no longer see patients as they walk in (or are carried in) from the street; no longer take detailed personal histories, no longer decide who will come into hospital, don't provide assessments or write discharge summaries, don't listen to people's problems and, very often, don't even listen at all. They are paid handsomely, of course, hospital psychiatrists earn much more than I do in private practice, even though I run a business and pay my own insurance and pension fund, etc. But what do they do to earn these breathtaking salaries? I don't know. If I ring a mental hospital, I can't talk to the psychiatrists. I have to talk to the triage nurse or the operations manager, the intake coordinator or even the allocations clerk. It reached its nadir when I rang a hospital to ask for a discharge summary on a patient I had sent to them, as the patient had been discharged and was told to come back to see me. "Yes," the receptionist said, "you can have it but the fee is $20.00 for us to get his file from records and then $1.15 per page for photocopying, plus postage and it could take two weeks because it must be approved first." Didn't they have an electronic copy they could email to me at no cost and no delay? "Definitely not," the woman snapped. All records had to be kept in a secure environment that met national standards of privacy and security and, until they had the patient's written authority on the correct form, they didn't even acknowledge his existence. Could I have a copy of the form for him to sign, as he was sitting next to me while I called? Most certainly not, they couldn't possible release a form, it was a legal document. I didn't bother: people who created and worked in such a dehumanized system couldn't possibly have anything worthwhile to tell me about the drugged man sitting mutely next to his frightened wife. Because this is the problem with the institution of modern psychiatry: there is no room in it for humanity.

Three decades ago, when I trained, psychiatry was exciting. It seemed to be moving ahead in leaps and bounds as the gigantic mental asylums were dismantled and long-term patients moved into smaller hostels in the community. With the right combination of drugs and psychotherapy, we felt we could help people back into real life. All that has gone now. Due to an utter failure of intellectual leadership, psychiatry has drifted from the mainstream and is wandering aimlessly in the eddies. Psychiatry is going nowhere and, while it drifts, everybody else who likes can take a bit of the body of the profession and run away with it. It is going nowhere because its leaders have no agreed model of mind to guide practice, teaching and research. Because it has no sense of direction, modern psychiatry focuses on the bits it can see: drugs and questionnaires, blood tests and brain scans. The notion that humans have feelings is ignored as being too squishy to waste time on. Bothered by feelings, are we? Don't worry, just take more of the purple tablets and come back in a month. You can talk to a counselor but if you start to cause trouble, we'll lock you up for the heavy-duty treatment. Next please.

Psychiatry has retreated from any concern about people as sentient beings just because it has no convincing model of mind that can grapple with the notion of suffering but, rather than do battle with psychologists and social workers over the souls of men (and women), it hides behind a facade of pseudoscience. Granted, the senior academic psychiatrists who set the pace, as they like to say, take umbrage at this, insisting that they have a genuinely scientific grasp of mental disorder. Why, they declare, we have scientific journals, we have congresses and university departments, we have degrees and gowns and prizes, we meet government ministers and have research budgets, committees and publication lists... surely you can't deny that this is what all other medical specialties do? Well, that's true, except for one crucial point: the rest of medicine has a genuinely scientific program to pursue. We psychiatrists don't: take away all the stuff and clutter of a "science of psychiatry" and there's nothing left. There is no program which says: This is the path to understand mental disorder. There is no agreed model to use as the basis of a science that cares about mental disorder.

If you want to test this, take any journal in any area of medicine and look at the first research paper that takes your eye. It will start with a statement of its position on a particular topic, giving references to establish its validity. You can then check the references, and the references they refer to, tracking back along the intellectual history of the topic until it reaches the most basic bioscience. A cardiology paper will lead back to the original papers detailing the elementary biological features of the heart, an orthopedic report will end with a skeleton and an account of the fundamental physiology of bone, and so on. But psychiatry doesn't. It will fade out somewhere in the distant past with some great man's assertion that "This is how it is." Quite often, it will be a pointless, hair-splitting argument over nosology, or some brave hope to find the final chemical cause of schizophrenia but what you will never find is how the paper fits into a larger, declared model of mental disorder.

Psychiatry has become a hollow shell in which the trappings of science conceal a pseudoscience. There are psychiatric journals, but not one of them addresses a declared model of mental disorder. This is why the profession is collapsing, this is why it can't attract the brightest medical students, this is why the average age of psychiatrists is rising and the average weariness of psychiatrists is so overwhelming that they simply acquiesce as yet another bit of the speciality is stripped away and handed to somebody who makes more noise. The greatest crime of the academic psychiatrists who are supposed to be leading the profession forward is that, having failed to deliver a formal model of mental disorder, they made psychiatry boring. That is why it is dying.

Perhaps this is how it should be. Perhaps we should take the Darwinian view that, if psychiatry had anything to offer, it would be thriving but if it doesn't thrive, then it shouldn't be kept on life support by legislation and government funds. Perhaps the psychologists and social workers and nurses and therapists and drug counselors and managers and accountants and lawyers are right: they can do it better. Perhaps they can, but I haven't seen any of them offer a valid model of mental disorder. It would simply set up more trouble for those who are least able to defend themselves. If nurses finally got control of the mental hospitals, then psychologists would soon demand their own institutions, then social workers and sex therapists, and so on. Instead of one mess, we would have a dozen squabbling empires, competing for funds and patients (in that order) and people in distress would still walk the streets at night because they can't find a mission statement that they satisfy. All this comes about because psychiatry has no formal, scientific model of mental disorder.

It is my view that, unless psychiatrists come up with a proper model of mental disorder as the basis for daily practice, teaching and research, then things will only get worse for the mentally-ill. This leads to an important point: Are there really mentally-disordered people out there? Or is the whole thing just a racket, designed to build empires and pay people to hide society's unfortunates?

I will argue on the one hand that any formal model of mind leads inexorably to the theoretical position that mental disorder should exist and, on the other, that it is an empirical fact that there are people who, by any definition, are mentally-disturbed through no fault of their own. Furthermore, I will draw in considerable detail the form of a suitable model, showing how it relates to philosophy, to the neurosciences and to common experience.

I-2. Summary of Part I: The End of Biological Psychiatry

It is the case that biological psychiatry is now in the same logical and sociological position as psychoanalytic psychiatry was in the 1970s. For decades, Freudian concepts dominated psychiatric thinking, especially in the United States. Gradually, however, psychoanalysis was coming under attack from a number of viewpoints. First, there was the historical evidence that a lot of what the early analysts claimed simply wasn't true. Secondly, major logical errors and inconsistencies were accumulating. Thirdly, there was very little evidence that it actually worked. From the late 1960s, psychodynamic concepts enjoyed a brief burst of popularity, a kind of agonal convulsion, especially from what was known as transactional analysis. This was psychiatry for the masses, mentalism for the mindless, and it generated an enormous industry in which everybody could diagnose himself or her neighbor (including children, don't forget "TA for Tots") and prescribe a course of treatment. It collapsed in self-parody, and psychoanalysis quickly slipped into well-deserved oblivion.

These days, we have a similar social phenomenon of psychiatry for the masses but the emphasis is biological. Every magazine urges its readers to tick the boxes and find out whether they have "clinical depression." TV advertisements urge viewers to call one of dozens of "hotlines" if they detect any deviation from psychic perfection in themselves or their families. Better still, "talk it over with your doctor who will prescribe the right treatment." School teachers badger parents to take their sons to pediatricians for "the tablets." Probation officers want their clients sedated until they complete their parole. Opticians frighten parents into buying spectacles to treat "central visual processing disorder" while every person charged with a crime claims to be the victim of a chemical imbalance of the brain. Antidepressants long ago passed antibiotics as the most commonly prescribed drugs. Everybody, it seems, is jumping on the biological bandwagon.

The worst thing that can happen to a science is for it to become popular. If couch potatoes can understand it, or think they can, then there is no hope. It says the theory is so simplistic that it probably doesn't even engage with its subject. In psychiatry, if every school teacher, social worker, psychologist, nurse, drug counselor, scout leader, chiropodist and neighborhood busybody can understand what makes people tick (a "chemical imbalance of the brain"), then they don't understand anything at all. This is because so-called biological psychiatry doesn't actually constitute a theory. Part I demonstrates this from several sides. Chapter 1 shows that biological reductionism is incapable of giving a rational account of human behavior. Secondly, the notion of there being but a single, physical cause of mental disorder is shown to be false. Finally, I use the example of the psychiatric publishing industry to show how the sociological phenomenon of modern orthodox psychiatry evades its primary responsibility as a science.

I-3. Summary of Part II: A Resolution of the Mind-Body Problem for Psychiatry

In fact, this claim is incomplete. What I do is detail a model which satisfies part of what we normally call mind, the part that is important for a theory of mental disorder. This develops the ideas first outlined in *Humanizing Madness*. Starting with common observation, I show how our concept of mind splits according to the "natural dualist" approach of the philosopher, David Chalmers. Next, his concept is applied to the work of the mathematician and logician, Alan Turing, which provides a conceptual basis for a cognitive theory of mind. At the same time, we have to give an account to what we know of the brain as a biological organ, and modern neurosciences are developing very rapidly. However, there is still a conceptual gap between brain and mind but it can now be bridged, and the concept of the logic gate fills the empty logical space between the mind as Chalmers envisaged it and the brain as modern technology is revealing it. Finally, we can move from brain to mind and back again without breaking any physical laws, without invoking the supernatural, and without denying our essential humanity. For want of a better term, I call this the "biocognitive model."

I-4. Summary of Part III: The Future of Psychiatry

This is perhaps anticlimactic: we can no more predict the future of psychiatry than we can predict the next hit song, or next week's Dow report. However, my view is this: that if psychiatry embraces either my biocognitive model or something like it, then it has a future. If it refuses, if it obstinately continues to chase after glib mirages, then it has no future. I don't know what would be worse, more bad psychiatry or no psychiatry, but I think a good psychiatry would be an improvement on both. Whether anybody believes that the biocognitive model is an improvement on what has gone before is up to them. My duty as a scientist is satisfied if I put the model forward for the new generation of psychiatrists, to look at, to use, to criticize, to improve, or perhaps just to discard for something better.

I-5. A Note of Thanks

I would like to thank the many people who have contacted me from around the world to offer encouragement. Dr. H. Keith Brodie, of Duke University, very kindly arranged an invitation to visit North Carolina, while Dr. Andy Kaufman surpassed himself with enthusiasm and hospitality. Prof. Michael Ruse, of Dept. Philosophy, FSU at Tallahassee, Florida, offered not just the chance to meet his post-grad students, but also his own hospitality. Prof. Alan Patience of Sophia University, Tokyo, provides constant encouragement. In particular, I want to thank my publisher, Mr. Victor R. Volkman, of LH Press, Ann Arbor, Michigan, for taking a punt on an unknown author from the far side of the world.

Part I:
Restricting the Scope of Biological Psychiatry

1 Defining Limits to Biological Reductionism

"If all possible scientific questions are asked,
our problem is still not touched at all."
Ludwig Wittgenstein

1-1. Introduction

The first half of the twentieth century was the golden age of physics. The second half, from the elucidation of DNA in 1953 to the description of the human genome, was dominated by molecular biology. Many people now believe the most exciting progress in the twenty-first century will be directed toward a rational account of the ultimate scientific mystery, the human mind [1]. From the psychiatric point of view, this will not come too soon. By a major measure of intellectual achievement, the Nobel Prize for physiology and medicine, modern psychiatry has had little impact. Even though mental health is the single most important cause of morbidity and secondary mortality in the world, there have been only two Prizes directed toward matters of psychiatry since they were instituted in 1901. Thus, when the author of a book entitled "Psychiatry, psychoanalysis and the new biology of mind," [2] is billed as "the first American psychiatrist ever to have won the Nobel Prize in physiology or medicine and only the second psychiatrist to have done so in the prize's 102 year history," psychiatrists may at last feel they are coming out of the shadows.

In this chapter, I will examine one author's concept of a single idea in psychiatry. However, the idea dominates modern psychiatry and the writer is extremely influential. Eric Kandel offers the view that "radical reductionism" will convert psychiatry and psychoanalysis into genuinely scientific fields. I will argue instead that reductionism is a restricted model of science which can never account for the entirety of human behavior, and can therefore never form the basis of a general theory for psychiatry. Furthermore, when applied to the field of human mental life, reductionism becomes incoherent.

1-2. Psychiatry and the Prizewinners

The first psychiatric Nobel award was in 1927 when the Austrian neuro-psychiatrist, Julius Wagner-Jauregg, was named for his discovery of the effects of malaria-induced fevers on the progression of tertiary syphilis, or general paresis of the insane. He had published his results in 1917 but his interest in the use of artificial fevers in treating psychosis dated from at least 1887, when he was attached to the university clinic in Vienna. He also worked on treating thyroid diseases and cretinism with iodine but this was long before modern biochemistry made accurate measurements of hormones possible. His conviction that fevers could improve psychotic states had no recognizable basis in the physiology of the time. It appears to have been an idea peculiar to his generation but he persisted with it long after everybody else had given it up. His major discovery was fortuitous, in that there were lots of people in mental hospitals with tertiary syphilis but, whatever the matter, Wagner-Jauregg's work is of no interest to psychiatry these days.

The next mention was in 1949 when Antonio Egas Moniz (1874-1955) was jointly honored for his work in psychosurgery. Egas Moniz was a Portuguese professor of neurosurgery who, remarkably, also sat in parliament and, as foreign minister, led his country's delegation to the Versailles conference in 1919. In the mid-1920s, after serving as ambassador to Spain, he returned to medicine and adapted the new techniques of contrast angiography to the brain, quickly gaining an international reputation for his pioneering work. In 1935, he attended a conference in London at which two researchers showed how cutting certain frontal tracts in chimpanzees' brains resulted in increased tractability. Intrigued, he decided to apply this to mental patients. The results of the initial series of twenty patients were considered encouraging and the procedure was widely copied. For example, in England and Wales, over 10,000 leucotomies were performed between 1942 and 1954. The figure was very much higher in the US but, with the advent of powerful tranquillizing drugs, people lost interest in psychosurgery and it soon fell into disrepute. The story of how the operation was championed in the US by Dr. Walter Freeman, and its tragic cost, is recounted in a recent biography [3]. Egas Moniz himself was not a psychiatrist. He was a neurosurgeon who applied his techniques to a psychiatric population, but not without penalty: in 1939, he was shot by a dissatisfied patient. A reviewer at the official website of the Nobel Prize stated: "I think there is no doubt that Moniz deserved the Nobel Prize" [4]. Today, very few psychiatrists would agree.

By contemporary standards, the work which led to these prizes would not meet the most elementary concepts of what constitutes reasoned research, let alone ethical conduct. Thus, when one of the world's outstanding neuro-physiologists, whose work is of the very highest intellectual and ethical standards, opines that the brain sciences can lead psychiatry from its intellectual wilderness, he can be sure of a large and eager audience. In his recent autobiography [5], Eric R. Kandel, joint winner of the 2000 Nobel Prize in medicine and physiology, describes how, after graduating from medical school in 1956, he did a year's internship in a general hospital followed by three years basic biological research in the NIMH as an alternative to national service [2, p109]. He then undertook a two year placement as a resident in psychiatry at Massachusetts Mental Health Center, which is affiliated with Harvard Medical School.

At the time of his appointment, American psychiatry was almost totally dominated by psychoanalytic concepts. His description of his training in psychiatry shows how things have changed over the years: "We saw only a limited number of patients... In those days, residents did not work very hard..." He continued:

> "Few of (our supervisors) thought in biological terms, few were familiar with psychopharmacology, and most discouraged us from reading the psychiatric or even the psychoanalytic literature because they thought we should learn from our patients and not from books... We learned next to nothing about the fundamentals of diagnosis or the biological underpinnings of psychiatric disorders... a rudimentary introduction to the use of drugs... often discouraged from using drugs in treatment because... it would interfere with psychotherapy" [5, p153-155].

While in psychiatry, he was able to conduct original research in hypothalamic neuroendrocrine cells in goldfish but he subsequently "...left psychoanalysis because it was unconcerned with biology" [2, p387]. He did not sit his examinations and has never practiced as a psychiatrist. Eric Kandel's prize was for his basic neurophysiological research on sea slugs. While he is a renowned and esteemed member of the Columbia University Dept. of Psychiatry, it is stretching credibility for psychiatrists to claim that his award reflects credit on this profession. He cannot claim that his undoubted expertise in normal sea slug neurophysiology qualifies him as an expert on disturbed human minds, not the least because sea slugs don't seem to have much in the way of minds.

1-3. Psychiatry and Biology

Kandel's book consists of eight papers and essays published between 1978 and 2001, together with an introduction, an afterward and invited commentaries by eight eminent figures in the fields of neurophysiology and psychiatry. The longest of the papers is a joint review but the rest are Kandel's. The theme of the book is that "radical reductionism" will "transform psychoanalysis into a scientifically-grounded discipline." He looks to the brain-based neurosciences "...to create a unified view, from mind to molecules... (a) new biology of mind..." This "unified psychoanalytic and biological perspective" can provide "a new science of the mind" from which would emerge "...a great unification into one intellectual framework of behavioral psychology, cognitive psychology, neuroscience and molecular biology." The means of uniting the disparate fields of "biologic and psychologic explanations of behavior" is by explicating the "biology of human mental processes." In essence, this means using molecular and genetic biology to provide "a new level of mechanistic understanding," confirming that "the basis for the new intellectual framework for psychiatry is that all mental processes are biological..."

This credo is repeated throughout this particular book, as well as his auto-biography [5] and both of his large and highly influential texts [6,7]. Biological investigation of the brain will allow us to "...understand the physical mechanisms of mentation and therefore of mental disorders." He emphasizes that the proper means of investigating the mind is by reductionist biology. He sees no limits to the capacity of biology to explain human behavior: "All the behavioral disorders that characterize psychiatric illness... are disorders of brain function. The task of neural science is to explain behavior in terms of the activities of the brain." Biology can transform psychiatry and psycho-analysis, turning them into a unitary scientific endeavor.

He defines mind as "the complete set of operations of the brain." Without exception, this definition places any and all mental states squarely within the explanatory scope of the reductive biological sciences: "If the neural representation of a sequence like a birdsong can be successfully analyzed, why should a sequence like a sentence be, in principle, less tractable to a neurobiological analysis?" [5, p400]. This includes mental pathology, which will be explained at the same level of function as psychoactive drugs, namely subcellular chemistry: "...we will join radical reductionism, which drives biology, with the humanistic goal of understanding the human mind, which drives psychiatry." If drugs work at the subcellular level, then that is the level where the primary pathology lies [2, pxxii].

In the main, the commentaries are supportive although Steven Hyman, a neurobiologist, warned that knowing everything about the component parts of the brain does not explain the whole of the brain's output. This amounts to a statement that the mind is an emergent phenomenon which cannot be explained by reductionism. Judith Rapoport wondered whether it was appropriate to try to reconcile biology and psychiatry. The last paragraph of the major essay (p316) suggests that reductionism might not answer all questions about human behavior: "Some might believe that all that is scientific about the study of life is illuminated at all levels from the molecular to the behavioral by what we know about DNA. But others might believe that there are issues about what it means to be a living being that are really not explained by the most detailed account of DNA." This comment is not typical of the views in the rest of the book.

Essentially, Kandel's collection of essays expresses the hope that reductive biologism will lift psychiatry out of its doldrums, probably by a "super theory" of psychoanalysis. This optimism has been called promissory materialism, which is an ideological stance, not a valid empirical theory. It is materialism in the sense that it promises answers to the most profound questions about the nature and state of the universe, using only the evidence of the senses and elementary reasoning. That is, there is nothing in the universe that the senses cannot perceive, meaning nothing beyond matter and energy, each of which is sufficient unto itself and requires nothing more than itself for its existence. In this view, all materialism is promissory materialism just because it says: Wait a while, all will be revealed by the ordinary processes of enquiry (or, as we would now say, of science). Promissory materialism is a very easy doctrine to hold as it says we don't have to worry about any really difficult questions because, when a suitable technology emerges, they will all turn out to be a simple matter of matter and energy. Thus, any intellectual effort now will be a waste of time, if not completely barking up the wrong tree. Materialists often point to historical examples of how a widely accepted theory was shown to be nonsense by the march of science. Examples include the theory of phlogiston and the vitalism of Galvani and Bergson.

I don't trust promissory materialism. It presupposes empirical answers to the really difficult questions about life and experience when nobody has ever established whether those questions are susceptible to empirical analysis. The history of science shows that there have been enough mistakes over the years for the uncommitted to retain a deep sense of skepticism about anybody who claims that "science will deliver the goodies." Nonetheless, I would be prepared to listen to anybody who wanted to argue the case for promissory materialism, but that is the one thing materialists will never do: argue a case. Their doctrine is all about *not* arguing cases. Theirs is the policy of "Just you wait and see." Take Kandel's sentence: "If the neural representation of a sequence like a birdsong can be successfully analyzed, why should a sequence like a sentence be, in principle, less tractable to a neurobiological analysis?" If what he says is true, then this sentence is itself of the same order and nature as a bird squawking in a tree. His sentences might be psittacine, but I firmly believe there is something in this particular sentence of mine that, in principle, a parrot could never understand. In passing, it is worth noting that promissory materialists often present their case as a series of rhetorical questions, just as Kandel did. For them, the answer is blindingly obvious and doesn't need a response, as time will fill in the details. If only life were so easy....

However, assuming there might be some value in his plan, several questions immediately declare themselves.

1-4. Psychiatry and Psychoanalysis

First, of all the available theories of mind, why would anybody choose psychoanalysis?

Kandel's autobiography shows that his commitment developed very early in his career: "I entered medical school (in 1952) dedicated to becoming a psychoanalyst and stayed with that career plan throughout my internship and residency in psychiatry... I (was) convinced that psychoanalysis had a promising future" [5, p44, p155]. Yet, despite his unrewarding experiences as a training resident in the early 1960s, his emotional commitment remains as fresh as ever: "This decline (in influence) is regrettable, since psychoanalysis still represents the most coherent and intellectually satisfying view of the mind" [2, p64]. He does not indicate that only a tiny minority would now hold this view [8,9]. He repeats the old error that Freud wrote a "metapsychology" (he actually wrote a metaphysical psychology) then suggests that, while "(w)e do not yet have an intellectually satisfying biological understanding of any complex mental processes..." a biologically-rejuvenated psychoanalysis might provide it [2, p67-9]. This juxtaposition of uncompromising reductionism and irreducible metaphysics is logically flawed.

A closer reading of his most recent works indicates an unreconciled tension between biologism and the belief that humans are something rather special. As his autobiography makes clear, Kandel retains a firm religious commitment. Throughout his scientific work, he repeatedly insists that biology will eventually explain the mind yet he does not indicate how biology can explain whatever it is that religions celebrate. If the expression of religious beliefs is a matter of mind at work, and the whole of the mind can be reduced to matters of genes and proteins acting at the synapse, then where does God fit in? I suggest his long-standing interest in psychoanalysis is a way of saying: "...and yet I believe there is something more to us than just chemicals."

He might argue that this is taking things too far but the justification lies in his own work: "An ultimate aim of neuroscience is to provide an intellectually satisfying set of explanations, in molecular terms, of normal mentation, perception, motor coordination, feeling, thought and memory...(and)... neurological and psychiatric diseases" [2, p193]. In a paper entitled "Genes, Brains and Self-Understanding," delivered in 2001, six months after his Nobel award, Kandel stated: "We already know that not only psychiatric disorders but almost all long-standing patterns of behavior—from wearing bow ties to being socially gregarious—show moderate to high degrees of heritability" [2, p381]. Because religious expression is unquestionably a "long-standing pattern of behavior," he must therefore believe that it will necessarily be explained by reductive biologism. However, since belief in God is a central part of many organized religions, especially Abrahamic, it inevitably follows that belief in God can be *explained* "in molecular terms." This case can be generalized, in that every living person has at least one belief which he or she regards as absolutely fundamental to daily life. It may be religion, politics, cosmology, anything, but the essential point is that, even at great personal cost, the individual will claim to hold it as a moral question, i.e. of freely choosing between right and wrong. There is, however, no conceivable, non-question-begging, deterministic model of freedom of choice. It is on this point, which we can call the 'supreme belief' test, that all biological models of mind will founder: either the person concedes his most prized beliefs (religion, politics, football club, scientific reductionism, etc.) are a matter of genetically-determined brain molecules, and therefore not his moral choice, or he must accept a non-biological model of mind, meaning reductionism can't explain everything about humans. They can't have it both ways.

This is not to deny that intraneuronal molecular changes occur, because they are the basis of brain activity, but where is the evidence that these changes are primary, that they have no prior cause? Biological psychiatrists assume they are primary but never bother to prove their case. I am no more convinced by the all-embracing claims of today's biological psychiatrists than I was convinced by the all-embracing claims of earlier generations of psychoanalytic psychiatrists. As it happens, I do believe there is more to human mental function than "mere molecules swirling in the dark" [10] but it is *emergent*, i.e. neither supernatural nor reducible. The prime mover in mental life is, as a natural phenomenon, prior mental events. That is, the arrow of causation in mental life goes from the mind to the brain, which is not what naive reductive biologism requires. Information processing by the brain constitutes a causative entity, above and beyond "mere neuronal activity," which augments the brain's computing capacity by many orders of magnitude. This gives us a mental ability vastly exceeding that of the great apes, even though our brain capacity isn't that much more than theirs. By this means, there can be beliefs that are not just "matters of genes and proteins influencing the synapse." This saves the moral basis of religious beliefs but immediately contradicts the reductionist "new biology of the mind," which requires that all beliefs must be explained in molecular terms. In short, the reductionist position is self-contradictory. Answering the next question may show why it is so widely held.

1-5. Psychiatry and Reductionism

The second question is this: Why reductionism?

Asking a committed biologist this question will evoke much the same incredulous stare as asking, say, "Why oxygen?" That is, to a biologist, the answer is simply common sense but, in such fundamentally important matters, common sense isn't enough. Richard Dawkins defined a philosopher as somebody who doesn't take common sense for an answer, meaning somebody who looks for the systemic faults in the standard view just because he is sure there will be some. These days, reductive biologism is certainly the standard view. Biological psychiatrists claim that the same physical explanation of the output of a bird's brain will necessarily account for the totality of the human experience. I disagree: while reading this commentary, your brain is functioning at levels which are in principle irreducible to the biology of an avian brain responding to a territorial call. Claiming otherwise, as Kandel does, is a misapplication of the principle of reductionism.

To answer the question, "Why reductionism?" we have to go back in time.

At the end of the medieval era, usually taken as the fall of Constantinople in 1453, mankind's place in the universe was fairly secure, if not always comfortable. As creator of the unvarying geocentric universe, God was omniscient, omnipresent and all-powerful, as well as jealous, vengeful and interfering. His special creation, man (with some doubt about woman) was positioned halfway between animals and angels. Knowledge of the (male) god-head was delivered to a select clique (of men) by divine revelation. Kings ruled by divine right, implementing divinely-inspired laws (as it suited them). Knowledge of the natural world had been revealed to semi-mystical figures during some heroic age in the distant past so that a medieval education consisted of ever-closer readings of the ancient masters. Daily life included a malevolent supernatural world in which the devil and his consorts lurked behind every tree. Diseases such as the Black Death were divine punishment which could only be propitiated by further torture and executions, usually of the most vulnerable in the society (e.g. women past breeding age). Life was, as Hobbes gloomily noted, "solitary, poor, nasty, brutish and short."

With the awakening of intellect we now call the Renaissance came a revulsion against superstition. Some of the most original and creative thinkers in history questioned the received view of the universe and realized the ancients had it all wrong. In 1543, two major but unrelated events occurred which are generally taken as the beginning of the Age of Reason. On his death-bed after a lifetime of diligent work, Nicolaus Copernicus published *De revolutionibus orbium coelestium.* On the other side of Europe, after a short but brilliant career, the youthful Andreas Vesalius published the equally momentous *De humani corporis fabrica,* after which he left the world of anatomy for good. These monumental works showed convincingly that anybody who wanted to know about the natural universe should start by looking at the universe itself. At an accelerating pace, revelation was replaced by deductive reasoning, while orderly observation took over from disputatious reinterpretation of the classics. In about 1597, the astronomer Johannes Kepler declared his ambition "...to show that the machine of the universe is not similar to a divine animated being, but similar to a clock." By 1616, Galileo was able to argue that examining the heavens themselves would reveal the underlying geometric rules governing the motion of planets. These general laws would eventually yield a further set of rules by which human behavior could be determined. However, the new breed of scientists didn't have it all their own way, as Galileo wrote to his colleague: "My dear Kepler, what would you say of the learned here who, replete with the pertinacity of the asp, have steadfastly refused to cast a glance through the telescope? What shall we make of all this? Shall we laugh or shall we cry?" (I have never found the original reference to this; it may be an urban myth).

Under the influence of such thinkers as Boyle, Bacon, Descartes, Newton, Leibniz and so many others, the revolutionary concept of a coherent and general scientific program gradually took shape. Its objective was to show that the universe was not a "universal mystery" but was a rational place, essentially a vast machine governed by laws which humans could discover by their own efforts. This program was the exact opposite of ideas that had dominated European intellecttual affairs for well over a thousand years. An essential part of the new rationality was to dispense with superstition, the idea that there exist entities and forces which can interfere at will with the natural world yet are not subject to the same rules as mortals. But once the process started, it could not be stopped. Soon, theism was replaced by deism, the notion that God could be discovered by reason rather than revelation, and that, while he had created the world, all he did was set in motion the rule-governed cosmic machinery then sat back, distant and uninvolved. From this point, it was but a small step to atheism, the actual negation of the idea of a Creator.

On the human level, philosophers argued that the body was a machine of exactly the same order as other animals. Humans differed from the beasts of the field only in respect of having an immaterial soul. Accordingly, the nascent scientific program was directed at explaining the basis of the bodily machine. Harvey's discovery of the circulation of blood, the development of the microscope, etc., soon showed that practically everything the ancients had said was simply wrong. Perfection did not lie in the past, it lay in the future, and would be revealed by human efforts, not through secret conclaves of bishops meeting among the musty tomes of jealously-guarded libraries. Since the body was a machine, its activity would be shown to be a matter of mechanics, of things acting on each other in accordance with the laws of motion etc., which the new thinkers were determining by reason and experiment.

Because they had no other conceptual models, the corollary to the new approach was that, where there is no magic in human affairs, there must be mechanism, i.e. rolling back magic revealed mechanism. Mechanism is properly examined by dismantling the machine to its component parts and seeing precisely how they interact with each other to produce observable behavior. This is called reductionism, the two-fold notion that larger things can be shown to be "merely" clusters of smaller things assembled according to standard physical laws, or that the behavior of complex beings can be shown to be the law-like outcome of the behavior of less-complex entities acting in concert [10]. Given the universal laws of nature which disciplined enquiry was already yielding, reductionism states that a proper understanding of the function of larger bodies flows exclusively and inexorably from knowledge of their microstructure.

It would probably be fair to say that reductionism has been the single most successful intellectual program in human history. Indeed, its many modern applications are increasing exponentially, even explosively. As success breeds success, researchers have widened the scope of the reductionist program to the point where they now see no limits to its explanatory power. As Kandel explained: "I spelled out my belief—almost a manifesto—that to understand behavior, one had to apply to it the same type of radical reductionist approach that had proved so effective in other areas of biology" [4, p236]. "Indeed, the underlying precept of the new science of mind is that *all* mental processes are biological... Therefore, any disorder or alteration of those processes must also have a biological basis" (p336, his emphasis). This emphatically states that there is *nothing more* to human affairs than "mere mechanism" in the form of molecules, genes, chemistry, etc. It positively excludes a controlling non-physical element which cannot be understood as the outcome of the same types of processes as govern, for example, the replication of viruses, or putrefaction. It states that understanding how the brain acquits its myriad functions which, collectively, we call the mind, is pure chemistry, mere push-pull, key-in-lock physical causation at the molecular level. Is this true? If a detailed knowledge of the microstructure of some large bodies accounts for the whole of their output, is this necessarily true of all large bodies, or do some defy reductionism?

1-6. The Limits to Reductionism

My case is that attempting to stretch reductionism to this point forces it beyond its natural limits. It is just this notion that causes biological psychiatrists to stare in disbelief: the idea that reductionism has limits, that it can't explain everything in the universe. I suggest the widely-held idea of '*reductio ad infinitum*' has arisen through an historical mistake, that of believing that anything that cannot be explained by push-pull mechanism (and sub-cellular chemistry is very much of this nature [6,7]) is necessarily mere superstition. Flushed with success, biologists have come to believe that there are only two sorts of explanation in the universe, theirs (the good sort), meaning everyday physical causation, or the bad sort, meaning magic. It is worth recalling that, at first, Newton himself had the greatest difficulty accepting the concept of gravity because it implied action at a distance, which was the hallmark of magical thinking. He could only think in terms of straight mechanics or straight magic.

This leads to another test which, with respect, I will call 'Newton's Apple Test': for any question of control, can we conceive of a natural "Third Way," a causally-efficacious alternative to mere mechanics and the supernatural? In brief, do we need to abandon our current models of explanation because they are restricting our intellectual development?

The natural limit to scientific reductionism is just this: it does not apply to anything controlled by some factor more than mechanism or "mere physical causation," specifically, the processing of coded information. Thus, a computer cannot be reduced to "mere chemistry" because there is more to it than chemicals. It has a program which, while actualized by tiny physical changes taking place in the machine, is nonetheless something more than those changes: it is driven by a higher logic than that of simple mechanics. Physical changes at a molecular or even subatomic level in the computer are the mechanism or agency of its data processing, but they are not the explanation. Psychology, which aims to explain human behavior *in toto*, is more than the sum total of chemical changes occurring in the brain at the neural or subneural level. Of course the brain runs on chemicals: psychology doesn't deny that, but its goal is to discover what controls the chemicals. While chemical changes in the brain are the mechanism or agency of belief, they are not the explanation. Further, since psychology has a physical substrate, there is no such thing as disembodied information processing, i.e. by developing a materialist alternative to mere mechanism, we can positively exclude the supernatural, which solves Descartes' classic problem.

Once we move into the area of belief, etc., reductionism is out of its depth. There is a crucial conceptual disjunction between the rules or laws of mechanism, which govern matter-energy interaction in a time-space matrix, and the rules of logic, which determine truth and falsity and thence meaning, value, etc., in a semantic (virtual) space. Mechanism and logic are not continuous but occupy different conceptual fields: as part of the material universe, matter is governed by the laws of thermodynamics whereas logical operations are not. By definition, matter cannot stray from the material universe to any immaterial realm (such as the semantic) and back again. This would breach the laws of thermodynamics because they do not apply in the semantic realm. Symbols, of course, cannot stray into the material realm because physical objects have no meaning. This argument applies to and negates any theory that tries to equate matter and mentation. I also suggest that the widespread and erroneous belief in unlimited reductionism is at least partly based in a semantic confusion. People seem to think that, because there are "higher order" laws, such as laws of the land or laws of logic or of chess, they will necessarily translate into the "lower order" laws of physics. This is incorrect: the "laws of physics" aren't laws in any formal or logical sense, they are mathematical relationships.

Kandel's concept of "radical reductionism" therefore cannot complete his projected program for psychiatry. He might object to this conclusion on the basis that his theoretical approach can account for the whole of mental life by another means, that of identifying mental function with brain function: "The basis for the new intellectual framework for psychiatry is that all mental processes are biological, and therefore any alteration in these processes is necessarily organic... Demonstrating the biological nature of mental functioning requires more sophisticated methodologies (than the microscope)" [2, p47-8; on p50, he hedges this slightly]. This amounts to Mind-Brain Identity Theory (MBIT), which states that mind and brain are identical. MBIT was popular in the 1950s and 60s but has since lost favor. The reasons are quite clear: identity is an absolute relationship which does not admit degrees. Quite apart from the small problem of thermodynamics, mind is not and never can be identical with brain, just because there are attributes of mind that are not also attributes of brain, and vice versa. The following example will show where MBIT breaks down.

Assume a neuron is in a specified physical state which causes the neuron's owner to be in a certain mental state. After the subject has a particular experience, that neuronal state changes in a slight but very specific way which alters its firing pattern, thereby producing a new mental state. Based on Kandel's own work, our present understanding is that the change is mediated by altered gene expression leading to the production of proteins which would otherwise have been suppressed. MBIT states that the new mental state is specific to just that change and to no other, and that any further changes in the physical state will necessarily result in a different mental state. However, we know that the body is in a constant state of biochemical flux—that, because of the endless turnover of metabolic components, the physiological state is never the same even from one minute to the next. Thus, the new protein molecules will eventually be replaced by another set which, while chemically indistinguishable, are not identical. They could also be replaced by other, quite different chemicals as long as they had the same properties, or even two neurons that did the same job as the original one. That is, the chemicals' role in the continuing expression of the new mental state is determined by their function, not by their physical state. Specifically, there is a relationship between the new mental state and the new function which the physical state subserves. But any relationship between the mental state and the physical state is contingent, not necessary. The mental state is capable of multiple embodiment, meaning primary mental control must vest in the brain's functional state, not its physical state. As physicians, we implicitly accept this point but it is precisely what MBIT says cannot happen. MBIT breaks down the moment we try to apply it to the human body as we now understand it. Can it ever be saved? I don't believe so. Like the theory of phlogiston, MBIT was proposed to fill an intellectual gap but was rendered obsolete by new facts.

To demonstrate using familiar examples, I can replace my computer while I am working on this paper but, as long as I save my material and install it on the new computer, I won't notice the change. The same goes for my brain. I remember things from childhood even though all the structures involved have been replaced a dozen times. As long as my body does its job, quietly repairing and replacing my ageing neurons, I am still the same person. Given the unique physical structure of the human brain, what counts in mental life is the brain's function, just because mental life is a functional state of the brain, not a physical state. This is axiomatic: the sentence 'The man bit the dog' uses exactly the same brain structures and consumes the same amount of energy as the sentence 'The dog bit the man' but has a totally different meaning. This is also true of many pairs of sentences, such as:

- One divided by zero gives infinity/ One divided by infinity gives zero;
- I saw a man-eating shark/I saw a man eating shark;
- All mental processes are biological/ All biological processes are mental.

In each case, the sentences are indistinguishable on the biological level, but their meaning is totally different. That is, they can only be distinguished by learning the codes, the conclusion being that the biological and the semantic elements in the sentences are not identical. Kandel's claim that "all mental processes are biological" [2, p47] is an attempt to bypass the really difficult questions in psychology by redefining them but it repeats the behaviorists' mistake: trying to expel from the field of science something that eluded their restricted methodology. The fact that the reductive biologists' methodology can't cope with the mind doesn't mean that the mind is a supernatural nonsense.

The goal of a reductionist "new science of the mind" for psychiatry, based wholly on the biology of the brain, rests on a fundamental error: the conflation of information and its physical substrate. Because of this error, the project will fail because it looks the wrong way along the arrow of causation. The historical basis of the reductionist error is the need to eradicate super-naturalism from our explanations of the universe. When it has explained the brain, its structure and how it perceives, manipulates, stores, recalls and transmits information, reductionism will have reached its natural limits because it will not be able to explain the information coded in the structure. Even when we can account for the disposition of every atom in the brain, we will still not be able to explain why humans have religious beliefs (or any belief). Beliefs are a complex matter of psychology. In turn, psychology is not determined by the laws of physical causation: what I believe is determined not by where those atoms are in my brain but what they are doing in the overall brain economy. And what the atoms do is decided, not by physical push-pull causality, but by my total informational state, by who I am and what I want. My mental state determines my brain state, not the other way around, otherwise we would be automata, like budgerigars chirruping at each other over their seed bowl.

Does any of this matter? I believe it does. There is no point abandoning a century of psychoanalysis and behaviorism because of their epistemological shortcomings, only to pick up another unproven '-ism' (in this case, biologism) and waste the next hundred years repeating the same mistakes. It is, however, worth asking why biologism has such a powerful hold on psychiatric theorizing. I suggest the reason is contamination of the notion of materialism by unstated religious yearnings.

Biological psychiatry appeals to people who want to believe in the soul, just because they cannot imagine the notion of a diseased soul. Souls come from God; they are created for the purpose and therefore have to be free of faults at the moment of creation. How, then, can such a perfect thing become diseased? Classic religious systems have no trouble with the idea of a willfully naughty soul and, in fact, base most of their ideas of human nature on this view. As they understand it, the soul sits inside the body, directing it in a state of full knowledge. But a mentally-ill soul is beyond comprehension, so the biological psychiatrists look to the body to explain the fault. It is not, they say, the soul that has broken down but the vehicle of the soul's intent, the reception point, as it were, from supernatural to natural. For example, I may speak to you by a faulty telephone line. There is nothing wrong with what I am saying but it comes out garbled at your end.

Furthermore, there is the Cartesian notion of a "unified, self-knowing subject essentially separate from reality but linked to it only by potentially deceiving sensory organs" [11, p77]. The soul sits inside its very imperfect vehicle, totally at the mercy of blurred eyes, addled ears, headaches and fevers. This saves the idea of the godhead's "perfect creation" but it sidesteps the really difficult question: How can there be a thinking entity which belongs to the natural realm? In discussing Nietzsche's contribution, these same authors commented: "...what get called truths are simply beliefs that have been held for so long that we have forgotten their genealogy." I suggest the idea of a perfect soul residing inside a very imperfect body is one of these "truths" with which people are so familiar that they don't even think to question it. But that is what philosophers do: they question the most basic assumptions underlying a particular belief system, happily mining them for howlers such as Kandel's claim: "The basis for the new intellectual framework for psychiatry is that all mental processes are biological, and therefore any alteration in these processes is necessarily organic... Demonstrating the biological nature of mental functioning requires more sophisticated method-ologies (than the microscope)." I submit that this is essentially incoherent.

Anybody who claims to hold religious views cannot also claim that those views, as mental processes, are biological in nature *unless* he is also claiming that there exists a soul which is not biological in nature, i.e. it is supernatural. This forces him to the view that mental disorder is due to a biological disturbance of the brain just because the alternative, that the soul itself is diseased, is unthinkable. Souls are divinely-created and have to be both seamless and incorruptible, meaning incapable of breaking down because, if they did, they would reveal themselves as being mechanical in nature as only machines can malfunction. If souls were themselves machines, then there would be no reason to suppose that they were not just natural products of the material realm. So people who take a religious viewpoint will necessarily be inclined to accept biological psychiatry, as Kandel did, just because the notion of a free-thinking, natural, mental entity that can break down implicitly threatens their religious beliefs.

Some people try to escape this quandary by taking the view that all mental disorder is just moral disorder, but their opinions also become self-contradictory when put to the test. I don't believe there is any evidence that panic-stricken people would endure their attacks if they had even the faintest idea how to stop them. The idea of mental disease as moral laziness has an immense appeal to those who have had the good fortune to choose their parents wisely, and their place of birth, etc., and have never stumbled on the path of life. They have clearly never considered the notion that mental disorder is a self-reinforcing trap that starts long before moral precepts have formed. I see their stance as a form of narcissism, and it is not worth taking seriously.

A theory of mental order logically precedes a theory of mental disorder. If we can explain how there can be a natural being capable of thought, then we will immediately be able to explain how it can malfunction. But because it is natural, we will also have shown how it can arise without divine intervention, which leads to the conclusion that immortality is impossible. A natural theory of mind explains mental disorder, but it also spells the end of received religion, and there are a lot of people who do not like that idea. That is why so many people are determined to prove that mental disorder just is brain disorder. They will not relent even if the attempt drags them into incoherence.

1-7. Saving Reductionism?

In their rush to label mentalism as supernatural, biological psychiatrists have overlooked a most important point: that it is logically possible for an empirical discovery to save part of their program. If somebody found that all mental disorders showed specific biochemical disturbances which were both necessary and sufficient for the development of the separate disturbed mental states, then the correct theory for psychiatry would be a restricted form of biologism [10, Ch.2]. However, this discovery would have nothing to do with a general theory of mental life: nobody could further claim that "all mental processes are biological," nor would they need to. The question of the correct theory of human mental life would remain wide open. The general principle is that, given any materialist system of mind-brain interaction, there is no logical necessity for a biological theory of mental disorder to be based in or derived from a larger biological theory of mind. Even without a biological theory of mind, there still can be a necessary and sufficient physical cause for schizophrenia but that is entirely an empirical matter. Biological psychiatrists have over-reached themselves by wanting to see their 'lesions' as part of a formal biological model of mind.

The crucial point here is that the larger theory (of mind) must be materialist because this provides the only guarantee that the diseased brain would cause a diseased mind (supernatural minds don't catch germs). Unfortunately, since materialist interaction goes both ways, biological psychiatrists would reject it because it also implies that some disorders would have a purely psychological causation. A wholly biological account of mental disorder could also become viable under the supposition of unidirectional interaction, specifically, from a supernatural mind to the brain. That is, given a supernatural soul or spirit which acts via the brain as its point of conjunction with the body, then, in the event of brain disorder, the spirit's instructions would become garbled in the transmission, somewhat akin to the effect of brain damage on the speech centers. However, even this possibility breaks down under closer inspection as it doesn't explain the central feature of mental disorders—that the sufferer's supernatural 'spirit' is in great pain.

I will also mention one more possibility only to dismiss it.

Panpsychism states that the mind is composed of lots of little bits of mentality that coalesce to produce what we experience as consciousness. Supernatural panpsychism says that the mental elements float around until they find a suitable lodging, which just happens to be the developing brain, where they merge. How they influence the brain, or what happens to them after death, is the familiar stuff of dualist philosophy and is not relevant here. A panpsychic naturalism states that the properties of mind somehow arise from matter itself, just as we accept that gravity arises from matter, but there has to be some significance in the organization of the matter, otherwise planets would be conscious. It has been suggested that organization is the clue, but this leads to the counter-intuitive notion that rocks and crystals, even cities or armies, have experience. Alternatively, the organization constitutes a machine, in the sense of doing work, but this model is indistinguishable from emergent dualism as outlined above. In any event, it denies biological reductionism because the properties of mind are, by definition, not those of the matter itself but are properties of how its organization works.

1-8. Conclusion: A Post-Reductionist Psychiatry

There is no convincing reason to believe that mind is reducible to brain but the main point surely is that biological psychiatry doesn't need that theory at all. A fully explanatory biological account of mental illness which is not embedded in or derived from a larger biological theory of mind is not self-contradictory. This does not commit us to spiritualism: while some people might like to see a supernatural soul as the director of the brain, a genuinely materialist theory of mind-brain interaction would render such a soul otiose. It would also avoid the logical inconsistencies of the reductionist approach. I don't believe there is any logical escape for a general biological theory of mental disorder, especially as we already have perfectly adequate psychological theories of causation of personality disorder, anxiety and depression, and of some forms of psychosis [10].

These days, psychiatrists show an intense ideological commitment to the biological program, yet a misplaced fear of being deemed supernaturalists (even if they are closet supernaturalists) prevents them seeing that their approach is fundamentally flawed. In order to temper the tidal enthusiasm for what is merely promissory materialism, it is appropriate to list the hurdles facing any biological theory of mind. I take this to mean "a theory that can account for the entirety of human experience wholly within the material realm of pure physical causality." Strictly speaking, this excludes any form of data processing but since some forms of data processing occur in all recognized nervous systems, we need to specify a limit. I suggest the limit should be set at the level of a cat brain, which allows the possibility that chimps and dolphins may have a restricted sort of mental life.

Within this limit, the minimal tasks of a biological theory of mind are as follows:

1. It must show how to generate an infinite output from a finite physical state;

2. Using insentient molecules, it must show how to generate sentience (sensation, emotion, cognition, etc.) without resorting to panpsychism;

3. It must show how complex systems of rules (such as football, banking, religion, etc.) derive from more basic rules such as the laws of physics or chemistry;

4. It must show how elementary physical entities such as molecules can generate symbols (including symbols of themselves);

5. Combining points 2-4, the theory must show how rules and symbols can generate language, in both its expressive and receptive forms, and other infinite and recursive symbolic and logical systems while remaining wholly within the finite physical realm;

6. The biological theory must give a coherent account of how molecules can generate predictions about the future, or fiction, fantasy, etc., and, of course, willful deception;

7. It must show how the laws governing particles and their interactions can act recursively to discover themselves without begging the question of a non-material mind.

I have already commented on the possibility of a biological account of mental disorder that doesn't depend on a biological theory of mind. Almost certainly, there are other important tasks for a formal theory of "mind as biology." Given these hurdles, one wonders why anybody would bother, especially as an emergent materialist theory of mind (natural dualism) can easily satisfy these requirements. For myself, I believe a biological theory of mind is a solecism whose appeal is predicated upon nobody trying to look beyond the slogans. Essentially, it is the modern equivalent of the geocentric theory of the universe, an easy solution to a profoundly difficult problem which is "neat, plausible and wrong." Reductionism is a restricted research program which will never yield a general theory for psychiatry just because it is the wrong conceptual approach. It would collapse if a viable mentalist theory became available [10]. It might say something about us when we recall that, of all the people in the world looking for the correct theory of mind, only psychiatrists still believe in reductionist biologism. As outlined above, I think the reasons for this fact are sociological, not rational.

The codes of the human brain that generate everything we call Mind are not available to a research program which, perforce, is confined to the physical realm of classic physics and thermodynamics. This is the null hypothesis: anybody who disputes it assumes the burden of proof. Oddly enough, and probably for historical reasons, biological psychiatrists thought theirs was the fall-back position, the point of least theoretical assumption. Yes, it is, but only if one denies the possibility that religion might mean something to the person who believes it.

2

Turing Computability and the Brain:
Critical Implications for Biological Psychiatry

> *"The popular view that scientists proceed inexorably from well-established fact to well-established fact, never being influenced by any unproven conjecture, is quite mistaken."*
> *Alan Turing.*

2-1. Introduction

The biological model is simply one of a number of approaches to the conundrum of mental disorder. Nonetheless, it must meet strict criteria before it can be considered a valid scientific approach. The goal of biological psychiatry is to remove all mentalist elements from our concepts of mental disorder, replacing them with biological constructs. These must have the same explanatory power as mentalism, yet remain wholly within the material realm and, *ipso facto*, be subject to reductionist explanation. I have previously examined two conceptual solutions to the problem, mind-brain identity theory (MBIT) [1] and biological reductionism [2]. However, neither theory could satisfy the minimal demands of a precisely-defined biological psychiatry. We cannot reduce psychiatric phenomena to the biological, replacing mentalist concepts with biological (non-mentalist) constructs, then trace the chain of causation back from (physical) atoms to, say, a sense of despair.

This chapter outlines an objection based in a completely different point of view. My case is that the central notion underlying the biological program in psychiatry [3] is defective, just because there are two potential explanations for any given mental disorder. Insofar as it has ever been explicated, the biological program in psychiatry requires that, for each and every mental disorder, there be a separate physical explanation which is both necessary and sufficient (i.e. unique and invariable) for that disorder. The explanation of each disorder has to be complete, with no need or room for mentalist elements to complete the chain of causation. However, I will argue that, in any explanatory system which integrates both the physical and the mental elements of life, every mental disorder can potentially result from either physical or psychological factors, yet the psychological cannot be reduced to the physical.

Deciding which is which is an empirical matter but, because of the fundamental nature of the brain as a calculating thing, the list of physical conditions known to cause mental disorders will never account for all cases of mental disorder. That is, there are and always will be mental disorders which are examples of pure psychological causation in a perfectly healthy brain.

Working wholly within a materialist ontology, the set of all potential causes of mental disorder, both physical and psychological, is always larger than the set of potential physical causes of mental disorder. It is definitely larger than the set of actual physical causes of mental disorder. Logically, it is possible that the set of cases of psychologically-caused mental disorder is empty but, empirically, we know it is not. Furthermore, there will be classes of mental disorder in which a psychological causation is both necessary and sufficient but, for any class of mental disorder, a physical cause can be at most sufficient, but never necessary. Any case of physically-determined mental disorder can be mimicked by one which has only psychological causes but not *vice versa*. This discrepancy of causation is inevitable and it is on this point that the biological psychiatry research program breaks down.

2-2. Turing's Universal Computing Machine

My case is based in the idea of the universal computing machine or, as it is now better known, the Turing Machine. It derives from the pioneering work of the British mathematician and logician, Alan Turing, who described the essential features of what we now call digital computers [4]. In Turing's time, "computers" were people who sat at desks and performed the calculations on which a mathematician's work depended. They had to follow standard procedures and were, in a sense, mere mathematical automata. Turing wanted to define the fundamental principles of a machine that could do the work of a human computer, but he extended his case to include the ideas behind any machine capable of performing any calculation. Initially, his interest lay not so much in building such a machine (he was later closely involved with constructing the first British electronic computers and was very familiar with the American work), but in defining the theoretical principles that are now taken as basic to all computing machines. Subsequently, after the first digital computers became operational, he proposed the general test which many people think was about testing machine intelligence [5]. It was not. It was his attempt at a rational (non-emotive, non-question-begging) response to the ancient question "Can machines think?" Apart from the title to the paper in which he addresses the question, he hardly mentions the word intelligence (or intellect, intellectual, etc.) in the paper (see Note).

Turing's legacy is based upon the notion of stripping the processes of computation to their essentials then devising a simple machine that can mimic them. He didn't attempt to write a theory of human intelligence; rather, he reduced clever behavior to its most fundamental features, to the point where these features could be duplicated by a machine capable of performing only the same few operations over and over again. By working on the problem, mindlessly, blindly, with no thought (*sic*) of time, tiredness, boredom, etc., much as ants reduce an elephant's carcass to bare bones, the machine could, in principle, reach a point where nobody could choose between it and a human. If a machine can actually do what a human does, then who minds whether it can think? "... I believe that at the end of the century," Turing predicted, "the use of words and general educated opinion will have altered so much that one will be able to speak of machines thinking without expecting to be contradicted" (p442). The clear implication in the paper is that, even though we are not sure how humans think, machines are in principle capable of mimicking the outcome by a whole range of different means, and the outcome is all that counts.

While the mathematical sections of his lengthy 1936 paper, "On computable numbers," are still beyond most non-mathematicians, early in the paper, he describes the general principles underlying digital computers. In lucid, non-mathematical form, he outlines the three basic design elements of a digital computer, the store, the executive unit and the control. The store or memory, as we would now call it, is the repository of the machine's instructions and actions. The executive unit "...carries out the various individual operations involved in a calculation" while the control ensures "that these instructions are obeyed correctly and in the right order" [4]. The machine processes a tape or data flow in accordance with its predetermined instructions or program, acting repeatedly upon each element of a calculation until it completes the process—all without the benefit of intelligence as we like to use the term. This describes what he termed a discrete state machine, the most basic form of digital computer. Because of its limited memory, it can acquit only a small number of tasks, perhaps just one. At any time, it is functionally restricted to a single program of activity which has to be rewritten every time any change in output is needed. Since its memory may be mechanical, changing the program in the memory might even necessitate rebuilding the whole machine.

The output of a discrete state machine is restricted in that it jumps from one discrete output state to another with no alternative positions between them. Of course, the individual output states can be very close to each other, so that the machine might seem to have an analogue or continuous output, but it still functions in a digital manner. This points to an important feature of any discrete state machine: that its output just is a digital flow. Until it is connected to an effector instrument or organ, it doesn't amount to much. Furthermore, if connected to different effector instruments, the same data flow can lead to totally different observable outcomes. This point is often overlooked as we are accustomed to thinking of simple machines in terms of what they do, rather than, as I am suggesting, distinguishing between the central controlling mechanism and the final output state. The central controlling mechanism constitutes the discrete state machine. With different connections, the same discrete state machine can control oxygen flow during an operation, detonate a nuclear weapon or send pornographic email (terrorists, for example, commonly use mobile phones to explode their bombs). This point is of very great importance in biology. In human terms, the discrete state machine in the respiratory system consists only of the medullary respiratory center; it has nothing to do with the diaphragm or the other respiratory muscles. They are the effector organs and are functionally distinct from their controller.

Turing's major contribution to the theory of computing was to recognize that, if the machine's instructions or program were not built into its memory but were coded into the input tape itself, in the same form or language as the data, then even the most restricted discrete state machine could be converted into a machine capable of computing a range of outcomes. Given enough memory, it would be able to calculate any possible outcome, meaning it could therefore mimic any conceivable discrete state machine, i.e. it would become a "universal computing machine." Suitably programmed, such a machine would beat any human computer. It would therefore follow that, in his test (which very deliberately looked only at output states), it would be impossible to distinguish the machine from a human, in which case all argument over whether machines can think would fade away. However, in a theory of mental disorder, it doesn't matter whether machines can fool us, what counts is the notion that a machine with complex or universal computing properties can mimic a simpler one to the point where they become indistinguishable. It is on this point that the model of mind implicit in the biological research program breaks down.

2-3. The Brain as a Collection of Turing Machines

As a preliminary, we need to stop trying to see the brain as a single organ with just one product. It is not: it is a cluster of more or less closely related systems under a variety of controls. Some of these systems are "mere" discrete state machines in the sense that they can only compute a limited output, while others can clearly change rapidly from one system to another after the manner of a universal computer. For example, it is possible to disconnect the respiratory and other primitive medullary centers from the rest of the brain and they will continue to work perfectly well without any higher input, as in deep sleep, head injuries, anesthesia, etc. At most, they are under a small degree of higher control: nobody can hold his breath until he dies, or will his heart to stop beating. However, the higher level speech centers can rapidly switch from speech to music to laugher, etc. while the highest mental faculties can jump from mathematics to whodunits by way of warfare and seduction with the greatest of ease. There is a hierarchy of control from the least to the most complex centers, where increasing levels of complexity (in what we call higher centers) lead to increasing levels of self-control, but the higher levels cannot force a lower level to do something its biological structure does not permit.

A "higher" center of the brain, meaning one with a universal computing capacity, can mimic the normal output of any lesser center. For example, I can force myself to breathe calmly even when my body wants to do something else, but I can also breathe in an unnatural way if I choose (the easiest way to distinguish between organic and psychological disturbances of breathing or of cardiac rhythm is to wait until the person is asleep, when psychological factors no longer apply). With a few qualifications, a higher center can always interfere with the automated output of a lower center, and the more complex the level involved, the easier and more convincing this becomes. However, because they are discrete state machines, the only possible innate disturbances in lower centers are organic—their "programs," as it were, are hard-wired into their biological structure. Any organic disturbance is likely to be stereotyped and can usually be diagnosed by eliminating the potential perturbing effects of higher mental function.

The brain systems involved in the true mental disorders are not just the equivalent of the automated medullary centers. They are much more complex, and their normal function is controlled by higher centers. The crucial question is whether abnormalities in their functional output are due to local physical disturbances or are a normal response to an abnormal input from a higher center. However, we cannot test a person's emotional state by seeing what it does when he goes to sleep, because that eliminates the very factor we want to test. Since there is nothing distinctive about the emotional disturbances with which psychiatry is concerned (only their frequency and intensity), this leaves us in the difficult position of never being able to decide whether a disturbance is primary or secondary. That is, purely on observation, we cannot tell whether an emotional disturbance is primary (biological) or is secondary (induced by unknown higher factors). A biological disturbance can always be mimicked by activity in the higher centers. More to the point, purely on behavioral grounds, we could not tell them apart. We would not be able to say whether a given disturbance of a lower center (such as emotion) was necessarily due to a biological defect ("chemical imbalance of the brain") or whether it was being driven by some factors in the programs of the highest centers. This is the essence of the Turing test. In common terms, the "programs of the highest centers" amount to the psychological state or state of mind: some factor in the mind can compel what seems to be a disorder of biological function. The crucial question is, of course, whether the most complex brain centers are properly conceived as "universal computing machines," but I believe the empirical evidence is very strong.

The biological psychiatrist will, of course, argue that this dilemma could be resolved if somebody invented a super-scanner that yielded the most precise and detailed information in real time about every neuron in that particular brain system. However, this wouldn't work: even if the scanner showed a specific chemical change which was both necessary and sufficient for the diagnosis, we would have no way of knowing whether it was primary or secondary to signals from the higher controlling centers. Biological psychiatry demands that any specific changes in the brain must be primary. The scanner might be able to show that the changes in the lower center depended upon certain activity in higher centers, and that this in turn depended on other centers, *ad infinitum*, but there would be no way of breaking the infinite regress without resorting to a mentalist explanation. The argument might then be: "Who cares if they are primary or secondary as long as we can reverse them?" Firstly, I believe the patient would care, and rightly so. Secondly, suppressing the emotional response to disturbed higher input does nothing to solve the problem but simply puts it on hold. The patient need only forget or lose his drugs for the problem to reassert itself.

2-3. *Mens Insana In Sana Corpore*

Arguing from a different starting point reaches the same conclusion. I have previously shown that mental activity cannot be reduced to brain activity [1].

My case is that mental activity just is another realm, entirely distinct from but intimately related to the physical, yet it remains causally effective in the real, natural world and is therefore part of the natural world. I suggested a solution to the mind-brain problem cast in terms of Turing's model of machine-based computation (this is expanded in Part II). The psychological realm arises from and is totally dependent on its physical substrate, but is nonetheless a separate entity with its own rules and conditions. Furthermore, because the psychological or mental realm is part of the natural world, it is possible for things to go wrong (in the same sense that things can go "wrong" in the physical world, as a failure to achieve the normal goal, such as genetic diseases). This creates the logical possibility that errors in the mental realm can create disordered conduct even though the physical substance of the brain is perfectly normal. Pure psychological disorders are logically possible; whether they actually exist is an empirical matter.

The usual analogy is the digital computer, which has two aspects, the physical or hardware, and the programmatic or software. The physical integrity of the machine is necessary for adequate functioning of the software, but not sufficient, as the software can also contain its own errors. That is, because the software is a process, there can be imminent factors which prevent it achieving a particular outcome. This is absolutely elementary and is in no way contradictory of any empirical, rational or logical principles: modern children immediately understand the notion of software bugs. My computer has its equivalent of "pure psychological disorders." However, this does not answer the question of whether humans can.

Normal brain function depends, we would say, on its physical integrity, including transient influences such as temperature, chemicals, tiredness, pain, etc. However, normal psychological function depends not just upon the brain itself (*Mens sana in sana corpore,* a healthy mind needs a healthy body), but also upon its own internal consistency as a controlling program. That is, for the physical brain, there is only one level at which errors can arise. For the mind, there are two levels, where the second level is dependent upon the first. This means that errors in the first level are not just relayed to the second but are compounded or magnified. Complexity itself also increases the risk of failure, which is probably why psychological disorders are more common among humans than among the anthropoid apes.

As we move from the basic cerebral functions, such as respiration, to higher order or more complex functions, such as emotion, then to speech and finally to judgment, the level of psychological control increases [1, Part II]. Necessarily, the scope for errors of control increases *pari passu*. Thus, if a person presents with a disorder of a basal function, there is slight chance it is caused by psychological factors, and distinguishing them is relatively simple. At the other extreme of brain function, the most common disorder of judgment is what is called stupidity. A person may be very bright yet still show a remarkable inclination to make short-sighted, self-destructive or just plain stupid decisions. This is not chemical. Our entire social system is based upon the notion that every citizen ought to act rationally: we cannot plead brain damage every time we get caught speeding. However, as soon as we move to an equally mysterious part of human life, emotion, there is suddenly a vast social pressure to blame genes, neurotransmitters, diet, etc., for every deviation. That should be qualified: we only attempt to attribute to brain disturbance those deviations we don't like. People who get excited at a football match, political rally, religious service, pop concert, etc., don't have a chemical imbalance of the brain. If they did, we could solve the problem of extremism very simply, but it will never work because a difference of opinion does not amount to a mental illness.

Finally, in the rush to find the schizococcus, it is often overlooked that the mind-brain is remarkably plastic and can normally overcome the subtle types of damage that are considered to be causative of mental disorder. With its enormous processing capacity, the brain can often cope with significant cortical damage with little functional defect. This should not be confused with, for example, the very obvious effects of strokes, etc., which are caused by localized damage to output tracts. The efferent tracts are not part of the computing capacity of the cerebral cortex and there is little or no interaction between them. Damage to, say, a pyramidal tract is not damage to the higher center itself but is functionally akin to damage to a peripheral nerve. That is, the mind may be able to overcome physical damage to the brain whereas the brain can never overcome a primary psychological impairment. This reduces the correlation between brain states and mental states, further weakening the case for biological reductionism.

2-4. Conclusion

The goal of biological psychiatry is to remove the idea of psychological causation from our concepts of mental disorder. However, to be convincing, this program has to be more than ideology: a convincing case for biological psychiatry would involve a suitable explanatory model relating psychology to biology. Both the main contenders for that model, mind-brain identity theory and biological reductionism, have been shown to be inadequate. The conclusion is that there cannot be a full explanatory account of mind, including its disorders, within the physical realm.

This paper outlines a further, theoretical objection to a crucial assumption in the biological psychiatry program, that there is only one potential explanation for each disorder, and each explanation is necessarily physical. Because the brain has the properties of a universal computing machine, there are perforce two potential explanations for each disorder, one physical and one mental. By its nature, biological psychiatry cannot tell them apart but will always attempt to deny psychological causation. In the highest mental functions, physical explanations of disordered output fade into insignificance.

It is important to consider whether the biological program in psychiatry can succeed. We should never forget that psychoanalysis and behaviorism exerted huge effects over psychiatry (and the public perception of psychiatrists) yet, despite vast expenditure of time and money over decades, both these programs failed and are now considered historical curiosities. They failed wholly for epistemological reasons, i.e. they were logically incapable of delivering the results that, in their initial excitement, practitioners attributed to them [6, 7]. The historical parallels with the mass enthusiasm for the modern biological psychiatry program alone should alert the critical observer.

Note:

Turing's renowned test is not a test of machine intelligence, not the least because the notion cannot be defined sufficiently rigorously to satisfy the unconvinced. He was aware that, as fast as computing machines could overtake human performance, skeptics would change the nature of any test in order to retain a sense of superiority over machines. Thus, the test he proposed was not a test of machine intelligence, but was actually a test of human intelligence, regardless of how it is defined. The question it asked was not: "Can the machine act in an intelligent manner?" because machines certainly can do all sorts of clever things. Rather, it asked: "Is a human smart enough to tell the difference between a man and the machine?" Turing's test turns the tables on the interrogator, effectively negating the effect of intellect in the process. That is, it was not so much a test of how smart man or machine was, but who was smarter. It is the same as seeing which of two people is taller: we don't need to know how tall either one is to realize who is the taller. And in the process, I have referred to a machine as 'who,' which is exactly what Turing predicted, sixty years ago.

3 Science and the Psychiatric Publishing Industry

"On the contrary, Minister, there's all the difference in the world. Almost anything can be attacked as a loss of amenity and almost anything can be defended as not a significant loss of amenity. One must appreciate the significance of significant."
Sir Humphrey Appleby: p133, The Complete Yes, Minister

3-1. Introduction

The case against biological psychiatry is now overwhelming. The reasons are the same as those which finished psychoanalysis and behaviorism: despite the ceaseless propaganda from the self-interested, it could no longer be denied that logical flaws meant that none of these systems actually worked.

Without invoking mentalist constructs to "bridge the explanatory gaps," nobody will ever be able to explain the whole of human mental disorder using only biological methods. Further, the majority of mental disorder is caused wholly by psychological factors operating within a perfectly normal brain. The logical arguments that lead inevitably to this conclusion are so fundamental that the wonder is how anybody could have overlooked them. The field of science is supposed to be restrained and impartial but, when it comes to mental disorder, we have major figures making wild statements that they have never argued, and never could justify (it's not just psychiatry that suffers in this respect: everybody is an expert on crime, education and mental disorder). For example, Samuel Guze, one of the most influential of American psychiatrists claimed: "There can never be a psychiatry that is too biological." Eric Kandel, Nobel prize-winner in neurophysiology, announced: "Radical reductionism (can) transform psychoanalysis into a scientifically-grounded discipline." It will show that "...the basis for the new intellectual framework for psychiatry is that all mental processes are biological." Brain-based neurosciences will "...create a unified view, from mind to molecules... (a) new biology of mind..." Similarly, Maxwell Bennett, a founder of the Sydney University Institute of Brain and Mind who holds a personal chair in this major university, believes: "...what has gone awry in mental illness is due to abnormalities in brain function... when the mind goes awry there is a concomitant pathological change in the function of... the brain."

These claims are pure ideology, not science. Granted, they come with the full support of the drug industry and many community pressure groups (who often get their information from websites maintained by the drug industry) and even government-funded bodies. For example, just this past week, a Melbourne-based organization called The National Depression Initiative, whose shopfront is the ineffably lowercase *beyondblue*, has mailed to most homes in the country a little questionnaire for people to discover whether they are depressed and, if so, a fridge magnet butterfly reminding them to hurry along to their general practitioner (family doctor) who will fix the problem with a prescription. At what cost, we don't know, although the website beyondblue.org.au shows that the group will spend approximately $90million in their first ten years of life. We are already over eight years into the program and they have grown into a national depression, anxiety, phobia, PTSD, OCD and panic initiative. Sydney, of course, has its own Black Dog Institute for depression but theirs is serious and eschews fridge magnets.

In short, ideologues have taken control of psychiatry; propaganda has replaced genuine scientific enquiry and nobody is permitted to criticize the established view. Now supporters of the establishment may take exception to this, pointing out that, just like all other fields of science, psychiatry has journals and conferences and seminars etc. in which the results of research are subject to rigid appraisal and public discussion. So there's no room for ideology, right? This view is wrong because the entire psychiatric publishing industry is a charade. It is a hollow pretence at science just because it lacks the most fundamental feature of any field of science, a formal, declared model of mental disorder toward which the research is directed.

This chapter will look at this point in some detail, using material from the various psychiatric journals.

3-2. Psychiatry as a Scientific Discipline.

The standard view is that psychiatry is part of medicine, and medicine is an applied science, therefore psychiatry is a scientific field in its own right. Very few psychiatrists would question this conclusion but, from time to time, it is appropriate to question our basic assumptions to see if they still apply. I have previously argued [1] that all models used in psychiatry are invalid, meaning our field is no more than a protoscience. In particular, I have outlined a case against the attempt to explain mental disorder using biological reductionism [2]. Briefly, reductionism is the wrong conceptual approach to the question of human mental life. That is, the attempt to reduce mental life to matters of biology is ontologically incorrect in that it misunderstands the nature of mind. My view is that since we do not have a valid model of normal mental life, or mind, we are not in a position to begin to explain disordered mental life. If we had an adequate theory of mind, then a model of mental disorder would flow from it and, hence, the correct technology for investigating and treating it. But, uniquely in medicine, we have nothing like this.

This appears contradictory: how can there be a field of science without an agreed model of what the field is about? At first glance, psychiatry has the trappings of a field of science. It has highly-trained researchers working in dedicated centers supported by government and industry grants which are allocated according to ethical processes. It has training programs, examinations, conferences, committees of ethics and a large publishing industry. Grant procedures, courses etc. evolve but the publication of scientific research is so basic to our concepts that we rarely consider it, and it has hardly changed in a hundred years. Its original purpose may have been educational but, these days, its major function is essentially epistemological, a matter of what we can rightly claim to know. Even though its applications may be covered by patents, etc., all basic scientific research takes place in the public domain. Theories must be free of bias, and the only way of ensuring this is to allow others to follow the arguments and to repeat the research. If there is a fault, somebody is sure to find it eventually. Publication serves other ends, of course, but its epistemological function is to eliminate error. Errors are discovered and corrected simply by placing the whole of the program, theories and research before the critical audience of one's peers and the general public. Accordingly, every part of a field of science is open to challenge. Nothing is sacrosanct, not theories, models or methods, nor personalities, reputations or ambitions. The idea that a field of science can be immune to criticism is self-contradictory, just because criticism is the only way we know of eliminating error. Indeed, criticism is the very engine of scientific progress [3].

As with all fields of science, psychiatry must meet certain criteria before it can be taken seriously. These include an agreed model of mental disorder (a 'single playing field'), objectivity (a 'level playing field'), accessibility (an 'open playing field') and accountability (a 'public playing field'). In this chapter, I will examine the question of psychiatry's formal status as a scientific endeavor from two points of view. First, does it meet the minimum criterion of having an agreed model? Secondly, do we assign the proper weight to the value of criticism in ensuring progress in our field? If we do not have both these features, i.e. an accepted model of mental disorder subjected to constant, institutionalized criticism—then we fail to reach the minimal criteria of any field claiming to be scientific in nature. These criteria will be tested by examining aspects of the publication policies of the main English-speaking psychiatric journals. It will immediately be apparent that, not only do we lack an agreed scientific model of mental disorder, but our approach to exploring the nature of mental disorder breaches some of the most elementary principles of scientific conduct.

3-3. What Do Psychiatrists Read?

The publication policies of each journal are displayed in their respective "instructions for authors," which are now found on the journal websites. One major journal restricts access to this page to fee-paying members but its instructions are available in the hard copy. A PubMed search of the word 'psychiatry' on December 15th 2008 yielded 326 journals.

(i) Models: Of the major, English-language journals of general psychiatry still in print, not one nominates a model of mental disorder in its instructions to authors. The *Journal of BioPsychoSocial Medicine* comes closest to naming a model. This journal, from Japan, has the most prodigiously long and detailed instructions for authors of any journal but fails to nominate the model of "biopsychosocial medicine" on which it is based. It describes the topics it will publish, which encompass "...all aspects of the interrelationships between the biological, psychological, social, and behavioral factors of health and illness.... (It) emphasizes a bio-psycho-social approach to illness and health... all of which are associated with mind-body interactions." No model of mind, of mental disorder or of mind-body interaction is specified.

The remaining journals give either very little or no indication of the type of psychiatry they will accept. Most offer a broad description of their areas of interest but do not attempt to define them. For example, *Archives of General Psychiatry* "...strives to publish original, state-of-the-art studies and commentaries of general interest to clinicians, scholars, and research scientists in psychiatry, mental health, behavioral science, and allied fields. *Archives* seeks to inform and to educate its readers as well as to stimulate debate and further exploration into the nature, causes, treatment, and public health importance of mental illness." Similarly, "The *International Journal of Social Psychiatry*... publishes original work in the fields of social and community psychiatry and in related topics.... Social psychiatry as a branch of psychiatry deals with the social, environmental and cultural factors in the etiology and outcomes of psychiatric disorders as affecting individuals as well as communities." The mode of interaction of these factors is not stated.

Others are briefer: *British Journal of Psychiatry* "...publishes original work in all fields of psychiatry." There is no mention of a model. *Psychosomatic Medicine* gives no indication of the type of work it will accept or of a model of psychic and somatic interaction. The *American Journal of Psychiatry* publishes articles which are "...reports of original work that embodies scientific excellence in psychiatric medicine and advances in clinical research." The particular scientific model the research is advancing is not specified. For *Australian and New Zealand Journal of Psychiatry* (*ANZJP*), "The acceptance criteria for all papers are the quality and originality of the research and its significance for our readership." There is no mention of a model of mental disorder and, on this basis, nothing to restrict it to psychiatry. A request to the editor of the *ANZJP* to explain how his editorial policy would distinguish genuine science from rabid fanaticism has never been answered. A formal complaint to this journal's sponsoring body, of which I have been a member for nearly 35years, has been ignored.

The website of the Canadian Psychiatric Association (CPA) shows that the Association's first objective is "...to uphold and develop the biopsychosocial approach to the practice of psychiatry..." This leaves the CPA in a difficult position: it is committed to "upholding and developing" a non-existent model. It avails nothing to argue that the Association is merely supporting a watered-down biopsychosocial "approach" because that is even more chimerical. Moreover, if the Association's chosen model of mental disorder is a phantom, where does that leave *The Canadian Journal of Psychiatry* (*The CJP*)? According to its website, the *Journal* exists to publish "peer-reviewed scientific articles" including reviews, original research, debates on controversial issues and letters to the editor, all of which must contribute to scholarly debate. Any author can submit "...scientific articles related to all aspects of Canadian and international psychiatry." In addition, the editor commissions editorials, reviews and debates and publishes letters commenting on previous papers. At first glance, this is uncontentious to the point of being banal: just another psychiatric journal publishing routine scientific material contributed by established researchers. This is Kuhn's "normal science" in action [4].

On second glance, however, something is wrong: at no point in its Instructions for Contributors does *The CJP* specify an agreed model of mental disorder toward which the "scientific research" must be directed. The only suggestion is that reviews will address "a broad range of biopsychosocial topics." While this appears to commit *The CJP* to a model nobody has ever seen, the *Journal* evades this imbroglio by omitting reference to anything more substantial. Effectively, this means the CPA and its "flagship" publication, *The CJP*, are operating without scientific warrant.

This listing of spurious and unsubstantiated claims could be continued through the entire list of 326 journals but it would be unproductive: there is nothing to indicate that all these journals of psychiatry have the slightest agreement or, indeed, any idea about what constitutes a valid model of mental disorder. On this basis, a reasonable person could conclude that, in fact, psychiatry does not have a theory or model of mind, a model of mind-body interaction or a model of mental disorder. This alone would disqualify it from claiming to be or have a basis in science.

(ii) Objectivity: The question of objectivity is best answered by looking at the subject lists published by the different journals. It is immediately clear that the field is tilted heavily in favor of reductive biologism supplemented by statistical analysis. These two fields, of course, dovetail neatly in that a detailed statistical approach is used to delineate the various syndromes or surface markers for which biology will eventually find the specific underlying biochemical defects. A complete biological model would then be in a position to devise precise pharmacological responses but there is no evidence of such a model. Biological reductionism has been assumed to be true, but no biological psychiatrist has ever offered an explanation of what would be involved in proving the statement: as far as they are concerned, mental disorder just is brain disorder. There is practically no criticism of the dominant statistical/biological approach in the mainstream literature, and no effort to present alternatives.

A review of 1196 published papers and commentaries in *ANZJP* for the calendar years 1996-2005 showed that only seven papers were critical in tone. Four of these were little more than minor gripes, e.g. one psychiatrist complained in passing that not enough research is done on the role of religious beliefs in mental order and disorder (in fact, he is perfectly correct: biological psychiatry cannot account for religion). Of the genuinely critical papers, two came from overseas and one was mine, meaning a rate of criticism of 0.25%. A recent editorial in the *Journal of Psychiatry & Neuroscience* was entitled: "The neurobiology of human social behavior: an important but neglected topic" [5]. Unfortunately, the journal's index indicates it is likely to remain so. Either criticism is not being written, or it is not being published. Either way, it is not being encouraged, meaning psychiatry lacks the *sine qua non* of progress in science: criticism of the dominant model.

(iii) Accessibility: The psychiatric literature is not open to "all players." Objective (1) of the Canadian Psychiatric Association is "...to uphold and develop the biopsychosocial approach to the practice of psychiatry..." There is no mention of where this approach has been substantiated, or its relationship with the long-discredited "biopsychosocial model" [1, Chaps 6, 8]. The *Canadian Journal of Psychiatry* "...contains peer-reviewed scientific articles related to all aspects of Canadian and international psychiatry" which, in the editor's view, represent a substantial contribution to the "scholarly knowledge base." At his absolute discretion, the editor invites eminent psychiatrists to contribute editorials, reviews and debate pieces on topics chosen by the editorial board. Letters to the editor are restricted to comments on published material. In brief, the editor determines what Canadian psychiatrists will read and controls criticism of his choice. Furthermore, the current editor does not accept or respond to comments on *The CJP's* editorial policy. The *American Journal of Psychiatry* will only consider letters critical of published papers if they are received within six weeks of publication and they have space. Essentially, this restricts critical comment to subscribers.

(iv). Accountability: Very few journals declare a policy relating to disputed assessments of submissions, although *ANZJP* is perfectly explicit: "The Editorial Board reserves the right to refuse any material for publication... Final acceptance or rejection rests with the Editorial Board." In practice, this means the Editorial Board of *ANZJP* applies its undefined criteria of quality, originality and significance *in camera*. Their deliberations may be rational but, equally, they may not be. Nobody who is not on the Board will ever know, and the Board is chosen, not elected. Other journals are coy on this question although only a very callow author would think that meant their decisions are open to question. This would not matter if the reviewing process were blind, but it is not. Because of the wording of the introduction and the list of references, reviewers can easily work out where the paper comes from and who supports it. I have had one reviewer comment to me that he recommended publication of one of my papers the editor overruled him.

3-4. Prejudice Masquerading as a Scientific Psychiatry

3-4 (a). Psychiatry without a model.

Currently, no psychiatric journal in the world meets minimum criteria for a journal of scientific record. Of 28 prestigious journals reviewed, not one defined the model of mental disorder that guides its publications policy. They simply do not have a model but conceal this fact under high-sounding phraseology. In the main, editors merely describe their field without defining it: "All submissions to *The Journal of Clinical Psychiatry* should be relevant and interesting to practicing clinical psychiatrists. We strive to publish academically sophisticated, methodologically sound manuscripts geared more toward the practitioner than the researcher." Relevant, interesting, sophisticated and sound: this is strong support for the view that psychiatry is merely a protoscience, if that.

Since no editor in the world today can give a working model of mental disorder, it would be reasonable to assume an open-minded approach to the question of what actually causes mental illness; but this is not the case. Publications policies are heavily biased toward the unproven and essentially unstated biological model. As an example of the tilt in favor of biological solutions to psychological questions, consider the following case study. A paper criticizing the biological model was submitted to *ANZJP* in July, 2006. Even though it proposed an alternative, it was rejected with a form response but was later published elsewhere [6]. In August 2008, the Journal published a highly partisan paper on biological explanations of mental disorder, written by a renowned neurophysiologist with no medical training [7]. A letter criticizing serious logical flaws in this paper was rejected with no explanation beyond "lack of space" (the criticism was that the neurophysiologist's paper actually supported the case for mentalism). At the same time, a further paper criticizing the biological approach was rejected with no explanation (it has since been published elsewhere [2]). In November 2008, the Journal published a further paper from the same neurophysiologist, again advocating a rigid biological solution to mental problems [8]. Once again, a letter pointing out serious epistemological faults in the biological papers was rejected within hours of submission. Two further papers of an intensely biological orientation were published in short order from the neurophysiologist while letters criticizing each of these were rejected. Shortly after, three papers detailing the basis of a solution of the mind-body problem (now Chapters 4-6 of this volume) were then rejected without comment although the editor indicated he would possibly reconsider them if "compressed into one paper."

Thus, the publication score is:
- four very strongly pro-biological papers, total 44 pages of biased philosophy and opaque neurophysiology written by a non-psychiatrist;
- four critiques of those papers rejected;
- two original papers critical of psychiatry's biological stance rejected but later published elsewhere;
- three further papers describing the basis of a mentalist psychiatry rejected.

I believe that amounts to a *prima facie* case of a biased editorial stance but it is permitted by the editorial policy of the *ANZJP* which states only that papers must be of "significance" to the readers. If there were an accepted model of biological reductionism to explain psychiatric disorders, this might be plausible but there is not. Since not one of the four biological papers addressed a declared model of mental disorder, their significance to psychiatrists is questionable. In fact, few psychiatrists would be able to read these densely-written biological articles, let alone find the major theoretical errors which the editorial board and their personally-selected reviewers failed to detect.

There is nothing to stop journal editors publishing what they like. When a journal announces that it publishes "...original work in all fields of psychiatry," one might assume that the editors would take care to present a balanced viewpoint, but this would be unwise. Like all journals, *The British Journal of Psychiatry* has a particular style and authors soon learn to place their papers in order to maximize their chances of success. Broadly-worded policies give broad discretion to the editors to pick and choose according to their unstated interests: "*Acta Psychiatrica Scandinavica* publishes high-quality, scientific articles in English, representing clinical and experimental work in psychiatry. The journal acts as an international forum for the dissemination of information advancing the science and practice of psychiatry." Since this particular journal does not offer a preferred model of mental disorder, it cannot claim to be following a scientific publishing policy, nor can it point to a "science of psychiatry." That is, journals publish according to editorial prejudice, all the while claiming to have a scientific publishing policy, even though none of them can point to it.

3-4 (b) Conducting science by show of hands.

Editorial boards grant themselves full and untrammeled authority to publish material they like (or reject anything they don't like) by deeming it high-quality, original, significant, relevant, interesting, academically sophisti-cated, methodologically sound or any of the other terms which disguise the lack of a declared basis for their decisions. In practice, anything can be rejected for any reason, and no explanations will be forthcoming, even though what is scientifically important very often seems quite insignificant at first (e.g. radium fogging a photographic plate in a drawer, Kaposi's sarcoma in young gay men, the failure of the Michelson-Morley experiment, fossilized seashells on mountain tops, changes in finches' beaks from one island to the next, contamination of an agar plate with *Penicillium*, a growth of *Helicobacter* in specimens of primary peptic ulceration but not from secondary, etc.). This anomaly arises just because there is no mention anywhere in any instructions for authors as to what constitutes a correct model of mental disorder against which the "significance" of their original, quality research can be assessed. There is no yardstick, no set of scales, no acid test, just whether the Editorial Board think their readership should read it or not. Journals do not publish lists of papers rejected, and psychiatry has nothing like the *Journal of Negative Results in Biomedicine*.

I submit this is not science but is indistinguishable in practice from mere ideology or prejudice.

In practice, modern psychiatric publishing reflects only a tacit agreement that the mainstream knows what the proper model for psychiatry is and need not bother itself with trivial objections, where all objections can be deemed trivial. This shifts psychiatry from the scientific camp to being merely a manifestation of a sociological phenomenon, group-think. This is when a self-selected, inward-looking or closed group of intelligent but like-minded men is catastrophically wrong just because they see no need for self-criticism and reject outside criticism. The international financial collapse of 2008 is a choice example of groupthink, as were the nuclear arms race, behaviorism and psychoanalysis, to name but a few. Similarly, the heliocentric solar system, plate tectonics, asteroid impact and evolution were all once considered completely absurd by the mainstream, and each of these advances came from a total outsider. This is consistent with Thomas Kuhn's sociological analysis of science [4].

It is critically important for all journals to declare their theoretical stance so that readers can know exactly what it is they are being offered in the name of science. If editors do not nominate the exact model of mental disorder they regard as correct, and give their reasons for choosing it, then they leave themselves open to allegations of a prejudiced publishing policy, such as favoritism. Worse still, the lack of a declared model of mental disorder leaves the boards no conceivable defense to allegations of prejudice. If, prior to the event, they do not name a reliable process by which papers are selected, then they cannot nominate the process *post hoc* and claim they have been following it all along. This is why civilized countries do not conduct trials *in camera*, and why people cannot be convicted by retrospective legislation. The rules have to be set out in advance for all to see. As it stands, the different editorial selection criteria listed above license not just rational theorizing, but also self-deception, whimsy, prejudice, chicanery, anything. What they do not establish is a rational, transparent process by which authors can judge whether they have been dealt with fairly, and psychiatrists can know that what they are reading is scientifically valid.

3-4 (c). Pseudoscience and fanaticism.

Editorial boards do not have a model of mental disorder to use to assess "significance." Instead, they rely on an inchoate notion of psychiatry as something biological that will be revealed by rapid advances in neuroscience after the way is paved by minute statistical delineation of syndromes according to DSM. This is not science at all. Manifestly, the editorial process cannot separate science from pseudo-science. It licenses prejudice just because it is indistinguishable from applied ideology. The policy of publishing "quality, original papers of significance to the readership" would fit comfortably with any extremist group in the world. But it is not and never can be science because science is a progressive, self-correcting or self-improving process driven by criticism of the standard view [4, 9]. On a more ominous note, the various notions of "significance" or "relevance" lend themselves to distortion of the scientific ethos. The test of "significance vs. insignificance" is no more rational than, say, "superiority vs. inferiority" as it was used by the eugenicists to mask racial prejudice. It is a pure value judgment masquerading as an impartial, scientific decision, and all the more sinister because it determines how we psychiatrists deal with other people's lives within a system of quasi-judicial authority. It matters whether we tell people they have a "chemical imbalance of the brain" just because the assertion alone renders them incapable of responding as an equal.

This means that, in effect, the psychiatric publishing industry is operating without scientific warrant. This is a bold claim but the justification is simple: science is directed toward elucidating models and theories of the universe and all therein. If there is no model of mental disorder, the research takes place in an intellectual vacuum and there is perforce not science. So the first question for any psychiatric journal to answer is this: what are we talking about? When psychiatrists (and remember that I am one) claim they have a scientific understanding of mental disorder, what is the nature of the claim they are making? I take it they are saying their approach is more than merely ideology, fad or whimsy. In practice, we are saying we should have first go at mentally-disordered people while others, such as crystal gazers, colonic irrigators, exorcists or euthanasiasts, should defer to us. However, to be taken seriously (which includes being paid serious money), we need a justification, an unimpeachable claim to having a superior knowledge about the causes and treatment of mental disorder. In essence, this means that we must show we have an established model of mental disorder which is firmly based in rational, empirical science and that it is better than everybody else's. And that is precisely what the international psychiatric publishing industry does not show.

Some people may take this to be little more than hair-splitting on the basis that reputable journals accept only scientific papers, and everybody knows what "scientific means." That argument has no merit: among many others, Freudians and Marxists once claimed that their theories were scientific, but we now accept they were ideologies with little empirical content [9, 10]. Unless the research is directed toward a specific model chosen by a transparent process, subjected to intense criticism and open to rebuttal by anybody within or without the profession, then the claim becomes self-serving. Effectively, the editorial board is saying: "Yes, we publish only scientific material, but we alone decide what is scientific according to criteria which we do not reveal." There is a further risk in this stance, that anybody who criticizes the established view may be deemed a heretic. Designating opponents as heretics is, of course, one of the hallmarks of non-science [11]. However, by mentioning orthodox psychiatry and heresies in the same sentence, am I not taking matters too far? I don't believe so, for the following reasons.

First, original research papers are accepted or rejected according to whether they meet the editorial board's implicit understanding of what constitutes a science of mental disorder. Because we do not know what it means by "scientific psychiatry," this may mean no more than "like/dislike the paper." Worse still, because the review process is not blind, it may only mean "like/dislike the author." There is no point insisting that this would never happen because what we require of a scientific journal is that, by virtue of a transparent editorial process, it *could* never happen. Bias must be impossible, and the first step toward rendering it impossible is to declare the model of mental disorder the board uses as its standard.

Secondly, editorial boards choose the topics for their editorials, reviews and debates, and then decide who will write them. For example, the Instructions for Contributors for *The Canadian Journal of Psychiatry* are very explicit on this point: "Unsolicited manuscripts are not accepted." So, armed with its private perception of what mental disorder is about, the editorial board chooses the people it feels will best address the questions it believes important, then insists readers comment only on the topics it has chosen. This might still be a valid scientific exercise, except for one critical point: the process does not allow anybody to distinguish between verifiable scientific progress, and mere question-begging (i.e. assuming the truth of that which requires proof). In scientific publishing, the burden of proof is very much on the editorial board: they must show that what they are doing is valid beyond any conceivable doubt. As it stands, there is not just room for conceptual doubt about the selection process, but it would be perfectly reasonable to ask whether the whole matter is simply a case of the establishment looking after its own interests. A necessary but not sufficient step toward establishing the editorial board's impartiality is to name the scientific model of mental disorder it uses as its standard.

The problem of psychiatric publishing is a sociological phenomenon which, I suggest, arose through an historical error which has simply never been addressed. The present format for journals, in which a largely self-appointed editorial board reviews submissions *in camera,* arose in the late nineteenth century. In those days, journals served more to educate than to disseminate the latest research. Papers were submitted for review by a panel of experts who decided what would help their few hundreds of readers. These days, the people who decide what the readers will see are very often those in the profession with the strongest reason for maintaining the *status quo.* In psychiatry, papers are screened by the very people who stand to lose most if the dominant approach to mental disorder were suddenly overturned. Again, this is entirely consistent with Kuhn's approach.

Finally, journals often advertise their citation impact factors as though the figures conferred some sort of validity upon their activities; but this is not the case. The impact factor simply gives the average citation rate for papers in each journal for the two year period after publication. It is not a measure of validity, simply one of internal concordance, and one which is easily manipulated. Quoting liberally and favorably from papers the journal has already published increases the chances that one's paper will match the editor's unstated concept of what amounts to good psychiatry. Thus, there is a self-reinforcing process whereby successful authors quote each other and, of course, their own work. By selectively rejecting material that does not agree with their unstated apprehension of the model of psychiatry, and by their (invited) editorials, editors covertly encourage authors to focus on topics and submit papers they know the editors are likely to view favorably, which essentially means citing papers the editors have already approved. This distorts the scientific process, as Ioannidis and his colleagues [12, 13] have argued:

> "Science is subject to great uncertainty: we cannot be confident now which efforts will ultimately yield worthwhile achievements. However, the current system abdicates to a small number of intermediates an authoritative prescience to anticipate a highly unpredictable future. In considering society's expectations and our own goals as scientists, we believe that there is a moral imperative to reconsider how scientific data are judged and disseminated."

This sentiment is not new. Lord Rayleigh (1842-1919), president of the Royal Society, noted at its 1897 meeting: "The history of science shows that important original work is liable to be overlooked, and it is perhaps the more liable the higher the degree of originality."

There is one more point about the "impact factor" that is often over-looked: it does not distinguish between favorable and unfavorable citations. For example, Prof. Bennett's turgid and, in my view, completely misleading papers on the organic basis of psychosis have profited quite handsomely from my using his papers as examples of bad psychiatry. As a measure of scientific validity, citations are hopelessly inaccurate. Since I debunked it in 1998, Engel's spurious "biopsychosocial model" [14] has had far more citations than my expose itself. In July, 2007, there was even a conference to celebrate it at the (huge) Westmead Hospital in Sydney although I wasn't invited to put the contrary view.

3-5. Conclusion

In practice, the editorial policies of all available psychiatric journals retard the development of psychiatry as a scientific discipline precisely because those policies actively inhibit criticism. Science is about progress, where progress means an inherently self-correcting process affected by criticism of the *status quo*. Criticism of the standard ideas just is the engine of scientific progress: no criticism means no progress, which is how we differ from Galileo's examiners (and who remembers even one of them?). Because editors refuse to be held to a declared standard against which their decisions can be independently judged, criticism of their actions is rendered all but impossible. By refusing to accept criticism, by neutering the very process by which inherent bias is detected and corrected, our journals push themselves outside the boundaries of science. However, after looking through hundreds of papers chosen because they are "substantial contributions to the psychiatric know-ledge base," perhaps the greatest crime of the psychiatric publishing industry is that is has made psychiatry boring.

For the purpose of initiating a long-overdue debate, I repeat my claim: institutional psychiatry and its captive publishing industry are devoid of a formal, agreed model of mental disorder. This alone negates its claim to be a scientific endeavor but the error is compounded by the publishing industry's refusal to countenance criticism of its secret decisions. By a process of passive or active neglect, orthodox psychiatry misleads psychiatrists, trainees, other medical practitioners and professionals, tax-payers and other funders, the general public and, above all, the mentally-ill, into believing that it has the answer to mental disorder almost within reach. The psychiatric literature is a major means by which this deception is perpetuated. This, in my view, exposes all psychiatrists to allegations of scientific fraud, and denies them any conceivable defense.

Psychiatry needs to address this question as a matter of urgency. The first step is to agree upon a model of mental disorder, then devise means of ensuring objectivity, accessibility and accountability. Given the fact of electronic publishing, these deficiencies could be rectified in a matter of months, if not weeks. The technology is available; all that is missing is the political will among editors to sign their power away. Biological psychiatrists know their approach to psychiatry is intellectually bankrupt and could announce this truth on the evening news tonight. The trouble is, they haven't worked out how to stay in power tomorrow. Controlling the psychiatric publishing industry is a very powerful means of staying in power.

Part II: Resolving the Mind-Body Problem for Psychiatry.

4

The Case for a
Mentalist Psychiatry

"For this is the great error of our day,
that physicians try to separate the soul from the body."
Plato

4-1: Introduction

To the ancient Greeks, the heart was the seat of the soul; the brain served merely to cool the blood of excess heat generated in the heart. In the fifth century BC, Hippocrates of Croton determined that the heart was of lesser importance. Based on his observations, he argued that the brain was the center of intellect while the heart was no more than the organ of the senses. This view persisted for several hundred years until it was revised by the Greek physician, Claudius Galenus, to use his Latin name. Galen suggested that the vital element of the soul resided in the cerebro-spinal fluid contained in the cerebral ventricles. This was possibly the first recorded attempt to localize mental function and it was remarkably persistent. For the better part of fifteen centuries, until the early Renaissance, Galen's interpretations of Hippocrates' writings dominated thinking in the Muslim and Christian worlds.

It was not until nearly a century after the fall of Constantinople in 1453 that anybody made a serious attempt to challenge Galen's ideas but the revolution was slow in coming. It began when an unknown physician working in an isolated and backward medical faculty realized something profound about Galen's teachings: the master from antiquity didn't know any anatomy at all. Andreas Vesalius gained his medical degree in Louvain in 1537 and died at the age of fifty, but his major work was completed by 1543, before he had turned thirty. In a few short years after he moved to Padua, he challenged the orthodoxy as nobody had done before. Unlike the ancients, Vesalius was a superbly capable anatomist. Moreover, he was not fettered by the old prohibitions on dissecting humans. He placed great emphasis on two revolutionary ideas: that professors should do their own dissections, and that people should believe their eyes rather than the ancient texts. Despite quite intense opposition, he produced two remarkable illustrated texts of human anatomy, one for physicians and, most unusually, a smaller version for students. Perhaps he realized that, if he wanted to overthrow the establishment, he should not waste his time preaching to the self-satisfied.

Vesalius' work led directly to the profound insights of William Harvey who, by a process of experiment and careful critical analysis, showed that the heart was more of a pump than a sense organ. However, his major work, published in Latin in 1628, was suffused with what we would now call *vitalism*. Just a few years later (1637), the French polymath, Rene Descartes, reasoned that the heart was nothing more than a mechanical pump. The way was open for the recognition of the brain as the seat of intellect, emotion and will. However, Descartes didn't take this step in public. The Church had very clear ideas on the place of the soul in human affairs and he had no wish to incur Papal displeasure, as Galileo had done in 1616. Instead, he argued from first principles that the soul acted upon the brain through the pineal gland. It activated the body's muscles by physically pulling on them, using threads in the nerves that Vesalius had shown in such detail.

There is nothing magical about the human body, Descartes insisted, it is just a clever machine, no different in principle from any other animal. Any and all differences between humans and the beasts of the fields were attributed to the immortal soul. This is the basis of what is now known as the Cartesian model of mind, the notion of an invisible little person or homunculus who somehow rents the space between the ears and runs the show. Descartes didn't invent this model, of course, the concept is so old and so widespread as to be the "natural" or intuitive model of human function. Even in modern times, it pops up in various guises, and not only because there hasn't been much better on offer since 1637.

Once it was generally accepted that the brain is the crucial organ in behavior, arguments soon developed over how it exerted its influence. One school formed around the idea of localization, that certain areas of the brain are endowed with specific functions that are constant from one person to the next. In 1825, Gall announced that he had discovered where the "mental faculties" were located in the brain. With masterful aplomb, he showed where such qualities as the senses of justice, prudence and the matrimonial instincts were to be found. From this developed phrenology, the idea that shape of the skull accurately reflected the level of development of that part of the brain beneath it. Thus, the character could be determined "scientifically" directly from looking at the skull itself.

In 1861, the localizationist view was hugely reinforced by Broca's remarkably accurate delineation of the speech area. Very quickly, neuropathologists began to find clinical evidence to show that many cerebral functions were highly and reliably localized in the cerebral cortex. These included motor and sensory functions, hearing and vision, etc.. Shortly afterwards, Betz showed that the precisely-located motor functions were associated with certain giant cortical neurons (1874), while other researchers showed that, at the microscopic level, each area of the cerebral cortex was populated by distinctive types of cells. Scientific precision soon undermined phrenology's crudities and, before long, it fell into disrepute.

By the beginning of the twentieth century, the influence of the monumental work of the Spanish neuropathologist, Santiago Ramon y Cajal, led to precise cytoarchitectural maps of the cortex, the most famous of which was by Brodmann (1909). With the discovery of the cause of general paresis of the insane, it seemed that scientific neurology was the wave of the future.

At the same time, there was an opposite school of thought, derived not from pathology but from natural philosophy, or what we would now call psychology. This school proposed that mental functions could not be precisely located in the brain, that they were part of a much more complex phenomenon which, because it was in principle unobservable, could not be disassembled. It was entirely arbitrary to locate unseen "functions" in the physical brain. Using experimental evidence from animals such as birds and dogs, Goltz, Flourens and other investigators proposed that the brain is a single, highly plastic organ, all parts of which are equipotent. Complex functions emerge from the brain as complete entities, rather than being assembled slowly from crude subunits of behavior. Their ideas weren't as outlandish as some people now assume: one thing the localizationists couldn't hope to explain was the speed and complexity of the highest human functions. Also, anybody could lead them into disarray by finding new functions and then demanding they find a localized area for it. Inevitably, there were far more functions than there was brain substance to support them, and so they seemed to render themselves absurd. Finally, there was always the powerful influence of those who believed that humans weren't just clever animals but were unique and special in creation, that human mental function could not in principle be explained by reference to the brain.

In time, the 'anti-localizationists' gained support from the new discipline of behaviorism, which held that the physical brain wasn't so important after all, that observable behavior was assembled from subunits of behavior subject to their own laws, rather than being built from simple push-pull physical machines. At about the same time, Freudian psychoanalysis, while nominally medical in nature, had nothing whatsoever to say about brain structure. It soon seemed that very large parts of the human experience could be explained without reference to the brain at all. Indeed, the psychoanalytic movement accepted non-medical (lay) analysts from very early. As late as the 1930s, Lashley took a strong stand against brain localization but this was the movement's swansong: following the Second World War, the modern era led in the opposite direction.

The two extremes were, on the one hand, that the individual psychological functions could be precisely localized in the brain structure and, on the other, that the brain was functionally a uniformly or equi-potential organ. The modern view is that the truth lies somewhere in the middle. One thread of the resolution originated in the 1860s, with the work of the renowned British neurologist, Hughlings Jackson, although the significance of his ideas was not recognized until long after his death. Based on clinical observations of brain-damaged and epileptic patients, Jackson suggested that neurological functions are vertically organized throughout the central nervous system. Functions are constructed, as it were, by the integration of representations at different levels of the CNS. Accordingly, given the internal organization of the brain, those functions can be "lost" by damage at a diverse range of critical points in the CNS. The localization of a symptom cannot be identified with the localization of a function, which was not what Broca had decided. In modern terms, we would say that cerebral functions are distributed throughout the CNS in a complex but wholly predictable way. There is nothing random about neuroanatomy.

Another thread is to be found in the work of the Soviet neuropsychologist, Aleksandr Luria (1902-1977). Luria graduated as a psychologist in 1921 and quickly developed an interest in psychoanalysis. He is reputed to have corresponded with Freud. Subsequently, he studied medicine which, for his era, gave him a unique conceptual approach to the brain. During the Second World War, he played a central role in managing the millions of brain-damaged Soviet soldiers. Post-war, he continued his research until shortly before he died. Working in the tradition of Pavlov and Vygotsky, he developed an approach completely independent of the psychoanalytic and behaviorist models then dominant in the West.

His model of mental function was years before its time and is now seen as entirely consistent with the cognitive neurosciences. His last major work, *Higher Cortical Functions in Man* [1], is essential reading for any psychiatrist interested in relating brain and mind. It is ironic that Western psychiatry, which claims to be the vanguard, has been enthralled by non-science such as psychoanalysis, naïve biologism or Engel's three word mantra, "the biopsycho-social model." [12] A comparison with behaviorism or psychoanalysis shows that Soviet psychology was on a different plane to the Western yet, to our detriment, it was very largely ignored.

In brief, Luria showed that higher mental functions can be understood within a materialist framework, i.e., the behaviorist "black box" can be opened without necessarily invoking mythical entities such as egos or souls. Human cognitive and behavioral functions obey consistent rules of organization. He developed a standard nomenclature for the different cognitive subsystems that helps unravel their mysteries, showing that the same principles of distributed processing generate the output in a wide variety of neuronal subsystems. This term, "distributed processing," is of critical importance. It is the half-way point between strict localization and rigid anti-localization (i.e. equipotentiality).

One of Luria's most important principles is that behaviors are assembled in serial fashion by homologous integrative functions at different points in the neuronal circuits subserving them. The concept is not dissimilar to Jackson's view. Accordingly, a detailed knowledge of the internal cerebral anatomy is a *sine qua non* of an understanding of behavior, from the most elementary to the most complex. In the following sections, I will show how Luria's approach demystifies some of the many highly complex mental functions that Western psychiatry takes for granted—and then misuses.

First, however, I wish to establish a formal basis for a materialist theory for psychiatry. It will help to reiterate some of the points established in my previous publications. The purpose in doing this is to clarify every point or assumption in the chain of reasoning from our most fundamental observa-tions, right through to an account of the most abstruse symptoms in mental disturbance. There should be no misunderstanding of any point in the chain of causation of human behavioral pathology. A theory which has "missing links" or which relies on some vague, unstated intuition to bridge explanatory gaps is not good enough. We've had too many of them in psychiatry and all they've done is hold us back.

4-2: Why Brains?

4-2 (a). Fundamental principles.

In my previous work, I proposed several conclusions about theory development in psychiatry. Since these are absolutely basic to a proper understanding of daily psychiatric practice, I need to reiterate them.

In the first place, it has been argued that there cannot be a non-mentalist theory of psychology. Some people would qualify this by saying "theory of human psychology" but, along with Tolman [11], I do not dismiss the proposition that certain animals, perhaps even the laboratory rat, have some sort of mental life. This means that naïve reflex psychology, as a sort of glorified physiology, has had its day. What we need now is an epistemologically plausible psychology, or knowledge of the psyche, meaning a rational account of the mind in all its aspects. It also means that the mentality of mind cannot be "explained away" by the legerdemain of reducing it to non-mental events. This means there will never be a physiological (or biochemical, or quantum mechanical, etc.) theory of mind. Minds exist; and even though life itself may be no more than a self-perpetuating state of chemically-based, thermo-dynamic instability, the mental element of mind is entirely novel in the history of the world, perhaps even of the entire Universe.

Secondly, a naturalistic dualism can explain everything a supernatural dualism can. That is, if somebody's postulated supernatural entity can interact with the body, a natural, immaterial entity can do the same without needing to invoke the supernatural. However, we need a new definition of "natural" to encompass the idea of "immaterial entities." If a narrow view of science can't deal with mentalist concepts, then we need to broaden our understanding of science.

Finally, a new theory for psychiatry must explain everything but a few elementary facts but these should be kept to a minimum. It is permissible to leave parts of a theory unexplained as raw givens: even though we live in a physical world, nobody has ever explained time, space, matter or energy. To us, they are brute facts, presently incapable of further explanation, but that doesn't stop us using these concepts in our theories and in our daily life. By analogy, there will be features of mental life that parallel these fundamental elements of the physical world. But their relationships must be precisely defined, so that we know exactly how, say, the mental equivalents of matter and energy interact. This is not the same as invoking explanatory entities, such as ego and id, which are in principle not open to further explanation. It simply says: "These empirical facts are unavoidable but a full explanation will have to wait."

4-2(b). Observational data.

Any theory for psychiatry will be based on three classes of information, the first being the *subjective world of conscious experience*. This is the "inner television," the private, three-ring circus hidden in my head. While there have been many attempts to concoct theories of mental disorder which pay scant attention to the subject's inner life, the essence of any theory of mental disorder is that it must explain the point at which odd behavior becomes madness. Two people may show exactly the same behavior, yet it may be that one is sane and the other insane. The distinguishing feature of mental disorder is that it hurts. It is said that a fully-established panic is the worst sensation a person can experience and still survive. Granted the privacy of mental pain means it is not intersubjectively verifiable, it is nonetheless as real as anything else I can perceive. Subjective pain is the *sine qua non* of mental disorder, and any account of mental disorder that omits its central element has failed.

Secondly, we have the class of *observable behavior*. This may include field observations of individuals or populations, or interviews, questionnaires, etc. In this context, behavior also includes speech and other forms of communication. We are interested in everything humans do, the good and the bad, as infants or as adults, intellectual or emotional, and so on. In particular, we are interested in human creativity, because it distinguishes us so clearly from other life forms on Earth. A theory of psychology must be able to account for human inventiveness, including dissimulation.

Finally, there is the vast and rapidly growing field of the *empirical sciences*, with emphasis on the neurosciences and computer technology. The day is long-gone when someone could write a theory of psychology in complete, even willful, ignorance of neuroanatomy and physiology. For a naturalistic theory, the neurosciences provide a critical means of "triangulation," an essential factual base for emergent mental life: "black box" psychology is now a historical curiosity. Unfortunately, the field of cognitive neurosciences is expanding so fast that nobody could hope to do better than maintain a passing acquaintance with the more important developments. In fact, this is all that is necessary. Because mentality cannot be reduced to biology, the basic neurosciences aid theories in psychology. They never drive them.

4-2(c). The tasks of a general theory for psychiatry.

At the very least, a general theory for psychiatry must account for the following features of human life:

Developmental psychology: Adult psychology does not arrive intact on a particular birthday. From the apparent mindlessness of the neonate, it develops according to a clearly-defined path, to some extent keeping pace with the maturing brain but showing unexpected spurts in other ways. The end result of this developmental process has to be commensurate with what we know of the brain, of behavioral achievements, and so on.

The neurosciences: An adult psychology has to be consistent with normal brain function, and with neurological disorders. Apart from Luria's much-neglected work, no theory in psychology incorporates anything more than the most banal truisms about neurology. Even though learning theory relied on a biological account of behavior, the two fields constituted different realms of discourse. Psychodynamic theories, of course, occupy an entirely different conceptual space from the neurosciences, with no points of contact.

Cognition, or the processes subserving knowing. This is the informational realm which, over the last forty years or so, has ridden to supremacy on the back of the highly successful computational revolution. The cognitive capacities include intellect, memory, and other elements, all of which have such striking parallels in the field of digital data-processing and are intimately related to the basic neurosciences.

Action: What are we if we can't put our ideas into action? A person locked in his head by a stroke endures what most of us would regard as the ultimate torture. Ideas are fine but, if they can't act on the real world, they might as well not exist. A theory of human mental life must be able to explain the interaction of the mental and the physical realms, showing how information passes in both directions without degradation.

Perception, or conscious experience, is what sentient life is all about. I like to taste my food just because it feels good; I look at sunsets, not for any biological reason but because the colors are so beautiful while music has started revolutions without anybody knowing why. Snails apparently breed without an orgasmic experience but few humans would care to follow their lead. Similarly, pain might signal tissue damage, but its real significance lies in the fact that it hurts. Sensation is the ultimate private joy, and the ultimate private prison. Anybody who says it doesn't exist or is irrelevant invites ridicule.

Emotion: Rage, affection, fear, laughter: some we share with animals, some we apparently do not, but nobody can deny the significance of emotion. These are the most violent of the brute facts, the most tempestuous and the most exciting (that's a tautology: excitement just is an emotion).

Creativity: Ants build cities, birds migrate vast distances and chimpanzees use grass stalks to catch termites, but no other creature builds opera houses then blows them up with long-range ballistic missiles. We design toys for children, and instruments of torture for them when they grow up; we create perfumes and Zyklon B; we compose love songs and military marches… this is not just intellect at work, because computers have "canned intellect." It is an urgent, driving force that shows no signs of knowing its limits. While we can build thermonuclear weapons and hurl them halfway around the world with deadly accuracy, we still have trouble with the question of whether we ought to be doing that sort of thing.

Psychopathology is the ultimate goal for any theory for psychiatry. A general theory must provide a non-circular account of the nature and development of mental disorder, showing how it is distinguished from normality and from neurological disorder.

4-2 (d). Does the brain control behavior?

Let me begin with a proposition so basic as to be a truism:

P1. Human behavior is neither totally random nor totally stereotyped (i.e. it is subject to variable control).

This proposition is probably a truism because, if our behavior were either completely random or completely stereotyped, I couldn't have written that sentence and you wouldn't be able to understand it.

If we agree on this proposition, three questions immediately arise:
(a). Where is the locus of control?
(b). What is the nature of the controlling element?

(c). What causes the controlling element to fail?

The concept of reproduction provides a physical analogy for the scope of these questions. We could ask: where is the locus of control in reproduction, what is its nature, and what happens when it fails? The locus of control is the gene, its nature lies in the realization of information coded in the DNA molecule and, when it fails, we see a wide variety of chromosomal and other anomalies. Where once people saw acts of God, we now recognize translocation errors, etc.

The rest of this section offers answers to these questions. When we can answer the third question, on failure of control, we will have arrived at a theory for psychiatry.

4-3: Where is the locus of control?

In a materialist ontology, i.e. excluding theories of supernatural control, the controlling element in human affairs must be located either in the environment or in the individual, according to the following options:

4-3(a). Environmental control:

Option (i). In the extreme case, somebody might argue as follows: "Some omnipotent thing in the environment constantly relays behavioral instructions to each and every individual." The immediate objection is that this notion amounts to the supernatural. In addition, it is an infinite regress. I move my finger. According to this theory, the Omnipotent Thing caused it to happen. However, if I believe that electing to lift my finger causes it to happen, then the Omnipotent Thing must convey to me both the idea and the movement. But if I suspect there is an Omnipotent Thing, then it must convey to me the idea that it conveys to me the idea and the movement, *ad infinitum*. The notion is not worth pursuing.

Option (ii). "The environment is mindless, but environmental stimuli control human behavior absolutely." We can easily devise experiments to show this is false. As a theory of behavior, this fails as it will lead either to a non-mentalist theory, or else to Mind-Brain Identity Theory, which has previously been excluded. It cannot account for the subjective experience of mental life or for creativity, so it would not meet the basic requirements for a theory for psychiatry.

Option (iii). "The environment sends a barrage of signals (mostly neutral), from which the individual chooses according to his needs." We can object to this as it is not a model of external control: ultimate control rests within the individual, not the environment. It is, however, worth pursuing a little, as it was effectively Skinner's model. Skinner located control in a dynamic interaction between the environment and the individual's genetic endowment. By virtue of their biologically-determined responsivity, he claimed, the behavior of organisms is shaped and maintained by environmental reinforcement of their operant behaviors. No mental elements intervene in the causative sequence of events. In this sense, Skinner was a "hard determinist" [2]. He argued that real control rests with genetic and external factors, meaning that what we see as mental concepts are illusory. The goal of Skinner's radical behaviorism was to show that a genuine non-mentalist psychology had precisely the same explanatory power as mentalist ideas without the pseudo-scientific trappings. Thus, he claimed to have translated mentalist language into precise formulations which did not need a hidden homunculus to complete the chain of causation.

As previously explained, his program failed, and any attempt to copy its central notions is also bound to fail, for the same reasons. Skinner could not give an account of such basic features of human and subhuman behavior as play, aggression, nurturing and so on. When it came to complex human matters such as goals, values and language, his program floundered. At first glance, that is a bold claim because his later works, such as *Beyond Freedom and Dignity* [8], he seems to show just this. However, there is a flaw in his claim, which we can call the "Tosca ploy." In Puccini's magnificently dark opera, the heroine, Tosca, believes she has a promise from the dreadful police chief, Baron Scarpia, to spare her lover, Mario Cavaradossi. The young man has been sentenced to die by firing squad but, in return for Tosca's honor, Scarpia agrees that the execution will be a sham. The soldiers will have no bullets, so their firing squad will be only a "firing squad." As it transpires, Scarpia cheats the young woman in that his "firing squad" is a actually a firing squad: their bullets are real after all, so the opera ends with bodies thudding to the floor all round and everybody is happy.

Skinner does this all the time. He puts scare quotes around a mentalist concept, such as "threat," "intelligence" or "moral values," as though something vital were missing from his use of the expression, just as there was to be something vital missing from Scarpia's firing squad which meant it was only a "firing squad." But Skinner does a Scarpia and, while everybody thinks he is talking metaphorically, just because that is the old language his audience is familiar with, he slips the vital element back in so that his "moral values" actually do the work of moral values as we normally understand the term. That is, they complete the chain of causation by means of a frankly mentalist factor. Thus, a "threat" in Skinner-ese carries all the mentalist menace and portent of a threat in your language or mine, except everybody thinks it doesn't: they are fooled by the scare quotes. Skinner could not translate the mentalism out of common language. His sterile, behaviorist schema could not arrive at anything like the power of language so he gave up and invoked "moral values" when only moral values could complete the chain of causation. Like Scarpia, the moment everybody was comfortable with the idea of the real thing being gutted, he smuggled the vital bit back in. The Tosca ploy conceals the intellectual bankruptcy of Skinner's anti-mentalist program.

This exhausts the possibilities for environmental control of human behavior. The central ideas of determinism have been around for a long time. While they have never been as influential as the concept of free will, they pop up from time to time, dressed in modern jargon.

4-3(b). Individual control.

Option (i): Again, the extreme case is readily routed: "The individual is born with a complete set of behavioral instructions to cover all contingencies he will meet throughout his entire lifetime." This is patently absurd. To begin with, there isn't enough storage capacity in the human genome to control more than a few hours of the informational requirements of anybody's behavior. Secondly, I would have to hand to my children not only the instructions for their lives, but also the instructions for every one of my descendents, *ad infinitum.* Thirdly, this approach cannot take account of environmental events such as the weather which, within broad limits, is chaotic. Finally, the behavior of all humans would have to be coordinated, which implies a Superior Intelligence, which places the notion firmly beyond the purview of science.

Option (ii). "Most behavior is under broad genetic control, while the rest is biologically-determined by means of acquired (learned) factors; no variables other than the biological intervene in the causative sequence between stimulus and response." This is Skinner's program in another guise. While it may work for insects and, perhaps, pigeons, it cannot adequately describe the behavior of mammals. Also, it would depend on a non-mentalist account of goal-directedness, which no drive theory can provide [3]. Once again, critical elements of the human experience, such as creativity, are not brought to account by this type of model.

Option (iii). "Behavior is largely biologically-determined, with a small mental component to account for the rest." This is the end of the line for non-mentalist theories: once a single element of mental control is admitted to the causative chain, then there is no way of restricting it. Also, it would be pointless to suggest that, having made the evolutionary jump to mental control, there would be no biological advantage in exploiting the faculty to its limits. This assumes, of course, that mental control of behavior is biologically advantageous, a hypothesis that the arms race might yet prove wrong. In any event, this option merges with the next.

Option (iv). "Given broad, genetically-determined biological limits to behavior, final control of the individual is determined by mental factors." In my view, this is the correct explanation of human behavior. At the various levels of human function, from the most elementary biology to the highest intellectual achievements, there are different forms of behavioral control, each of which determines a different research program. One of our first steps is to decide how to approach each level: somebody might feel that fetuses decide the color of their hair post-conception, but the molecular theory of genetics provides a better account.

All living creatures have a great deal in common: we humans need food, shelter, partners and somewhere to care for our offspring, but so do crocodiles. We like to play, we are social and hierarchical, but so are dogs; we use tools, but so do chimps. Investigation of the broad limits of animal behavior is effectively a search for biological similarities. Psychology becomes an investigation of the narrow differences that count. We all need food, but why are some people prepared to share theirs while others are miserly? We need affection, yet some people shun society. We have urges to dominance, yet some people are submissive.

Option (v). "The entirety of human behavior is under mentally-mediated control." I mention this extreme case only to dismiss it. Hunger, coughing, pain, orgasm and waking are not under mental control in any meaningful sense of the term.

From this very brief consideration, we can conclude that human behavior is the outcome of an interaction of genetically-determined similarities and psychologically-mediated differences. Just which is which is an empirical matter.

4-4. The nature of control: mentalism vs. non-mentalism

It is clear that there are various modes of control in human behavior. First, there are such basic drives as the need for food, water, air, sleep, shelter and so on. There is little doubt that these are biological imperatives, but less clear are such matters as the drive for company, for sexual partners and dominance etc. Historically, the higher drives such as curiosity, the need to play and explore or fear of strangers, were assumed to be psychological but we now know that all higher primates show them to much the same extent as humans. It may well be that these have strong biological components, perhaps just as part of the maturational process, but psychological factors can easily interrupt them.

Thus, just like chimps, I have a biologically determined capacity for fear but I still have to learn what is safe and what isn't. The nature of a belief may be a matter of biology but the literal content of beliefs, etc., is entirely a matter of psychology. There does not appear to be any way for biological factors to intervene here: genes, as has often been said, code for proteins, not for ideas. Furthermore, there is insufficient genetic material to control the content of belief systems. Finally, as mentioned, there would be no biological advantage in a complex system such as mentality having evolved without using it to its limits.

This is not the right place for a detailed discussion of the research program into the biological basis of human similarities, or what we might call human nature. At the least, it embraces anatomy, physiology, biochemistry, molecular genetics, and developmental and cognitive psychology. However, an understanding of these subjects is essential in any attempt to understand human psychology, as psychology is intimately related to its biological constraints.

4-4(a) Non-mentalist psychologies

Behaviorists attempted to build a non-mentalist human psychology, but it is central to my case that this is doomed to fail. Broadly speaking, their position was as follows: As a materialist discipline, science can only be concerned with matters which can be publicly measured by objective observers. Thus, the mind, which is private and immaterial, is not the province of science.

Over the years, there have been many arguments raised against this strict positivism [e.g. 1,4,5,6], not the least being the rather telling point that, as psychology, it doesn't actually work. In his far-reaching attempts to derive a positivist psychology, Skinner [7,8,9,10] argued that "mentalist explanations" are not explanations at all. All they can do is posit an internal and unverifiable agent (a homunculus) which affects whatever it is that requires explaining. Apart from being invisible, homunculi have all the properties of humans and thus, in real terms, they explain nothing. Skinner therefore dispensed with all accounts of human behavior which invoke intervening mentalist variables, psychoanalysis being the best-known example. Ultimate causal efficacy, he insisted, is a biological phenomenon and all would eventually be revealed by physiology [7].

Dennett [4,5] took the opposite view, arguing that, in trying to dismiss mentalism, Skinner had made a very basic but serious error. Dennett was of the view that the psychologist had wrongly supposed that all mentalism was necessarily supernatural. He countered this by showing that it is not wrong to posit internal agents as long as they are eventually explained in material terms. Computer programmers and those working in artificial intelligence do this all the time and, provided they know that they will be held to account for their homunculi, there is nothing magical or intellectually dishonest in the ploy. Thus, Dennett removed a major part of the rationale for Skinner's anti-mentalism.

However, Skinnerian anti-mentalism cannot stand alone; it rests on other premises. If we deny the efficacy of mind, we must replace it with some other causally-effective agency. In the anti-mentalism of radical behaviorism, the adjunctive premise is the belief that behavioral events are wholly explicable in physiological terms, and therefore comprehensible in all respects by the methods of positivist science. The environment is the agency by which physiology gives itself the best chance of survival. If mind is causally ineffective, if all behavior is the outcome of (biological) brain events, and if all brain events can be investigated in their entirety by positivist science, then a complete understanding of brain physiology will explain all possible behaviors. If, for example, we want to understand what people say and why they say it, then we need not look beyond the physiology of the speech centers and a few other bits and pieces. Anti-mentalism depends on this proposition (or something very like it), but I believe it is wrong. My case is as follows.

Consider the example of somebody doing sums in her head. Since the human brain is capable of performing a potentially infinite series of calculation, we can only presume it is not "hard-wired" for arithmetic, i.e. there is neither a separate neuronal circuit for each and every possible calculation, nor even a separate molecule. Since many regions of the cortex are dedicated to functions such as vision, motor functions, etc., only a relatively small proportion of the cerebral neurons can be involved in performing mental arithmetic. That is to say, a finite part of the brain can produce an infinite output. Thus, those neurons involved in mental arithmetic must be used over and over again, just as the logic circuits of a desk calculator or the balls of an abacus can be used forever without once repeating a calculation. For a finite machine to achieve an infinite, non-random output, its processing activity must be coded. In the case of the neuronal "arithmetic centers," both the input and output are symbols (digits). Since this is a materialist (non-magical) account, I take it that the neuronal activity in these centers thus represents the symbols in coded form: the symbols themselves are coded into the brain's physiological activity but, being symbols, they are not identical with that activity.

However, we do not know the code the brain uses to perform its calculations. It follows, then, that the fact that a neuron is activated or involved in some process of calculation does not permit us to draw any conclusions about the significance it carries in that calculation. Its significance can only be understood in terms of its outcome. Without knowledge of the codes involved, knowing that a particular sequence of neurons is activated in a calculation will have no predictive value for us. Mapping sample patterns of activation will tell us nothing because there can be no direct correlation between a particular (finite) pattern of neuronal events and its (potentially infinite) output. Thus, knowing the pattern subserving the calculation (2+2=4) would not allow us to draw any conclusions regarding the neuronal events subserving the sums (1+1=2) or *zwei und zwei gibt vier.*

We can generalize this conclusion to cover all events where brain codes are used to manipulate the symbols used in generating an infinite output: if we don't know the codes, we can't know what the brain is doing. Skinner's theories depended absolutely on the notion that watching the brain in action will inevitably tell us what it is doing in the mental sphere. I conclude that his program could never have succeeded. The case against the positivist approach is further strengthened in that there is no reason to suppose that all brains are identical with respect to the positioning and connections of every particular neuron. In biology, normality consists of a range of values and the same principle must surely be true of the most complicated organ of all, the brain. Accordingly, if we know exactly what sequence of neuronal events happens in Mrs. Smith's brain which denotes: "I've been thinking it's Wednesday," we could never be sure that the same sequence will obtain in her brother. And what about "*Pom wah pen wan sook*"? (he lives in Thailand). In any event, how could we know all this without taking poor Mrs. Smith's brain apart? All this argues against the view that there can be a non-mentalist form of control of our behavior.

Another confusion which flows from the positivist view is that a complete knowledge of brain anatomy and physiology would allow us to predict all possible behaviors, just because there is nothing else that can affect behavior. Skinner, of course, was obsessed with the idea of "prediction and control." For example, if we fully understood the brain centers subserving speech, we should be able to predict all possible poems. If we understood the neurophysiology of humor and of speech, then we should be able to predict all possible jokes; of music, all possible hit songs; indeed, we would be able to tell the future of the human race, which would be helpful but isn't going to happen.

It may be countered that this is a little extreme. A Skinnerian may argue that a complete understanding of the immune system will tell us exactly how an individual will react to any particular infection, but it will not tell us which infections he will contract. That depends on his environmental contingencies, which is entirely in keeping with radical behaviorism. I don't believe this could constitute a defense. Firstly, while the immune system uses codes, it does not do so in any sense in which we use the term in connection with speech. The immune system depends on crude, 'lock-and-key' codes which have nothing in common with those subserving the transfer of information between individuals.

Secondly, knowing a person's past history of bacterial environmental contingencies would allow us to predict with great precision how the individual will react. But it doesn't matter how well you know my brain, your knowledge will never allow you to know why I laugh at something one day and curse it the next. In order to do that, you would need to know my brain codes, which you could only do by two steps. You would need to isolate every neuron in my brain and then test it formally against every possible environmental contingency, which is impossible on both counts. You would also need positive knowledge of every item of information I have stored in my memory (i.e., you would have to know everything I do know, and be sure of everything I don't know), which is fanciful (forget that it is possible in principle). The Skinnerian might counter that knowing the brain in question in all its molecular detail would reveal all this information, but my response is: How would anybody know what my brain knows without either asking me or without having some sort of standard measure, say, somebody else's brain? This is an infinite regress, and is therefore non-scientific.

The inductive methods of neurophysiology therefore cannot allow us to understand what is happening in the brain with any predictive certainty. Without predictive certainty, there can be no science, meaning there cannot be a non-mentalist science of psychology. We need to look for another means of tackling the coded brain activities which underpin symbolic behavior. This is not to say that physiology cannot deal with any codes at all. It has successfully worked out the genetic codes of DNA and the directional codes of bees' dances, among many others, but these differ from the example above in that they are finite and are symbolic in only a very direct and restricted sense.

We can conclude that Skinner's ambition to write a non-mentalist psychology could never be achieved. That is, his goal of understanding human behavior in strict biological terms, reducing language and other symbolic activities to simple matters of biochemistry, was doomed. The human brain stores and processes symbols in a physical substrate but these have a significance going far beyond mere matters of neurochemistry: the coded information is more than the brain events underlying it. The mind runs the brain, because if it were otherwise, our behavior would be stereotyped and entirely predictable and we would not have the intellectual wherewithal to analyze it. Stereotypy can never analyze creativity. There cannot be a non-mentalist psychology.

4-4(b) Mentalist psychologies

These arguments against non-mentalism amount to a sufficient case in favor of mentalism: our behavior is necessarily controlled by mental events just because any other explanation is either supernatural or cannot be taken seriously. I think this matter has to be seen in its historical context. Psychiatrists have spent the last century struggling to find a suitable model of human behavioral control. Psychoanalysis was a vastly influential but profoundly flawed attempt to give a formal, rational basis to the idea of mental control of behavior. It was flawed in that it could not be anchored to reality, which is why it drifted into the nether reaches of nonsense. Behaviorism, on the other hand, recognized that there were limits to the scientific method and restricted their field to observable behavior only. Both of these moves were legitimate, they just didn't work. Biological psychiatry is an attempt to fudge the issue. It says the mind exists and it is causally significant but it isn't really a mind after all, it's just chemicals which can be investigated using the methods we use to check feces.

It is time to move on. We need a mentalist psychology just because everything else has failed (remember Churchill's comment on his mother's people: "We can trust the Americans to do the right thing, but only after they have exhausted all the other possibilities"). Positive proof of a mentalist psychology will come only when we can define "mental events" with the certainty required to establish non-physical control. The fact that modern science cannot yet convincingly tackle mental events is not a reason to deny them. Instead, it is a powerful pressure to develop a better sort of science. As long as everybody is aware that all talk of mental events is provisional, that we need them to complete the causative chain before we can fully account for them, then no harm can come from it. The digital revolution shows that the idea of clever machines is not fanciful. Whether we can extend this case to humans, or have to develop a different approach, remains to be seen.

4-5. Conclusion

This chapter has outlined a case in favor of mentalist control of human behavior. It started with the most basic observations possible and progressed through a series of options to what seems to be the inevitable conclusion. The locus of control in human behavior resides in humans themselves, and its nature is mental, not biological. Mental events control our behavior, just because it could not be otherwise. Normal behavior is caused by mental events which are associated with or result from the processing of information coded in the brain. Thus, when we come to talk about the causes of mental disorder, the first place to look is the causative level of mental order. The remaining chapters in Part II will derive a mechanism by which mental events can control physical behavior.

This does not exclude the possibility that biological factors may contribute to certain mental disorders but that is an empirical matter. We do not yet have the technology to decide this question for any condition but, so far, the results are unconvincing. I don't see the point in spending another cent on the biological research program in psychiatry, especially when we have such strong reasons to believe that it will never yield the results its fervent supporters have always trumpeted are just around the corner.

5 Toward a Molecular Resolution of the Mind-Body Problem for Psychiatry

"Gravitation: the tendency of all bodies to approach one another with a strength proportional to the amount of matter they contain—the quantity of matter being ascertained by the strength of their tendency to approach one another. This is a lovely and edifying illustration of how science proceeds, having made A the proof of B, makes B the proof of A."
Ambrose Bierce, The Devil's Dictionary.

5-1. Introduction

The next task is to outline a causative theory of mind which can serve as the basis for a general theory of psychiatry. Even though we physicians are trained in the tradition of reductionist biology, and the dominant ethos in psychiatry is biological, we still believe there is something more inside the head than just a brain. That is, we secretly believe in what Gilbert Ryle called the ghost in the machine. One might say we are all closet dualists. I want to reconcile this ontological tension, between our public, biological faces and our private beliefs in favor of a form of dualism.

From the philosophical point of view, there is no point hoping that reductionist science will solve the big problems of psychiatry as, for example, it solves the big problems in infections, metabolic illnesses and genetics. That is, we cannot hope to "explain away the mentality of mind." As the philosopher, David Chalmers, often says, "We need to take consciousness seriously" [2]. Anybody who claims to have a non-mentalist theory of mind is making a claim that no-one in history has been able to justify. My own work starts with Chalmers' injunction and builds a foundation of a theory of mind for psychiatry, using only principles which have been clearly established in other fields.

5-2. Chalmers and Property Dualism

Previously, it was argued that the aim of a biological model for psychiatry (essentially, a non-mentalist theory of mind) derives from a profound mistake, that of believing that anything which is not frankly material is spiritualist, or even magical, and is therefore non-scientific. However, the concept of substance dualism is now so outmoded that it is little more than facile to criticize dualism on the basis that it necessarily implies magical substances: it is over 300 years since Spinoza outlined the notion of property dualism. Chalmers' contemporary version puts the case for a property dualism that "...gives us a coherent, naturalistic, unmysterious view of consciousness and its place in the natural order" [2, p165]. A brief summary of his case is given in Ch.10 of [1], so what follows is a summary of a summary of a major philosophical work,

It is necessary to take consciousness seriously: "The easiest way to develop a 'theory' of consciousness is to deny its existence or to redefine the phenomenon in need of explanation as something it is not" [2, p xii]. Consciousness is "a natural phenomenon, falling under the sway of natural laws," with the consequence that "there should be some correct scientific theory of consciousness." A complete, reductive explanation of consciousness is impossible. Physical theories will never tell us anything interesting about experience. Eliminative materialism is simply an attempt "...to evade the problem by denying the phenomenon" which need to be explained (p164).

Consciousness exists but, since it cannot be reductively explained, we need to develop a natural form of dualism. Even though naturalism denies supernatural properties, it is not to be taken as synonymous with materialism: "All that has happened is that our picture of nature has expanded ... (T)o embrace dualism is not necessarily to embrace mystery" (p 128). This contrasts with Daniel Dennett's uncompromising stance: "...dualism is to be avoided at all costs... accepting dualism is giving up" [3, pp33-37]. Chalmers proposes that conscious experience supervenes naturally upon the physical realm as the result of a series of psychophysical laws. These will transform a dualist theory from metaphysical mess to a comprehensible account of one of the most difficult concepts in nature. The laws, however, won't necessarily be capable of further explanation themselves: they are laws of nature, not of logic.

Critically, consciousness divides readily into two aspects, the realm of phenomenal experience and the psychological or cognitive realm. The former is the inner, subjective world, the compelling but ineffable sense of "what it feels like to be something." "Psychological consciousness" is the knowing, informational and reportable sense of self which I can convey to you by symbols. Unlike Dennett's functionalism, which tries to explain consciousness away, dualism was never meant to be easy.

With two sorts of consciousness, we get two mind-body problems and one mind-mind problem. There is the problem of contact between the body and the psychological self, between the body and the phenomenal realm, and between the psychological and the phenomenal realms. The mode of interaction between the psychological realm and the body is easy to grasp. There is nothing conceptually novel or difficult about transferring information between these spheres. The real trouble for dualism arises with the explanation of the nature of phenomenal experiences. For the time being, these are left as brute facts. Conscious experience is not yet (if ever) capable of further explanation.

Despite their differences, the two realms of mind are closely related. Every time there is a conscious experience, there is also a related psychological assessment or phenomenal judgment about that experience: "...information is the key to the link between physical processes and conscious experience" (p 287). "A conscious experience is a realization of an information state; a phenomenal judgment is explained by another realization of the same information state" (p 292).

Thus, there is no convincing logical reason why we should deny that humans are creatures with dual-aspect, insubstantial minds in their heads. If we broaden the notion of materialism to include the concept of information processing, and allow that the mind arises from, or maybe just is, the high-speed manipulation of data by a very, very powerful biological data-processing machine, then we have the basis for a theory of mind which will satisfy psychiatry's need for a natural, dualist-interactionist model of mind. But first, we need to consider the tasks of any theory of mind: what do we want our model to do?

5-3. The Tasks of a Theory Of Mind

5-3 (a) What does the mind do?

A theory of mental life has to account for a wide range of phenomena. These include:

> **(i)** Exteroceptive sensations such as sight, sound, smell, touch, pain, temperature, position and vibration sense, pressure, sexual sensations, balance;
> **(ii)** Interoceptive sensations such as hunger, thirst, tiredness, nausea, loss of breath;
> **(iii)** Emotions such as anxiety, anger, joy, humor, sadness, etc.;
> **(iv)** Compound emotions such as triumph, despair, suspicion, novelty and familiarity, guilt, yearning, awe;
> **(v)** Cognitive functions such as knowing that and knowing how, calculating, deciding, working out, judging, recalling, being aware of, believing, intending, hoping for, expecting, realizing, meaning, implying, deceiving, getting a joke, detecting injustice, taking a hint, taking offence.

Of course, it is one thing to give a theoretical basis for these functions, something else again to show how these functions influence observable behavior. How does the insubstantial mind act upon the very substantial body? That is the classic mind-body problem, and I propose that a solution to this problem is within reach. First, we need to define mind in such a way as to make it amenable to a conjunction with the physical realm, which was the problem Descartes outlined 350 years ago.

Of the mental phenomena listed above, the first four groups (i-iv) are brute facts which can be experienced but cannot be further analyzed: they can only be defined ostensively. Empirically, they fit very well with Chalmers' description of the experiential realm. This is the feeling, experiencing aspect of life which, for most of us most of the time, seems to dominate existence. Ordinarily, when people speak of the mind, they have 'in mind' the constantly active and interactive internal screen or arena that is stuffed full of vital experiences. Experience is so much part of us that we take it for granted, yet the very act of experiencing something seems like one of the great miracles of the universe. That there is life is remarkable; that we can perceive it and reflect upon it confounds us.

The other class, of cognitive or knowledge-based functions, is entirely different. These are not experiences but are processes or executive functions which occur outside awareness. Their only point of similarity with conscious experiences is that they all occur in the head. The cognitive functions are fast, reducible, communicable (as information) and silent (unconscious), in that they have no experiential content and are not open to introspection. We do not know how these come about, as we are not privy to their processes; we are simply appraised of their results. Thus, we can never catch ourselves in the act of making a decision. We can think about lifting an arm but the instantaneous decision is forever a mystery: we can never catch it in action. Similarly, I don't consciously decide this thing is a human face: that knowledge is provided *gratis* by processes I can never see in action. I don't know how I catch a ball or tie a necktie, but I'm pretty good at it. I can walk and talk and do crosswords without giving these complex activities a moment's thought. Now if there is any meaning to the word 'unconscious,' I suggest it is this, an unconscious processing of the information on which life depends. Splitting something into its parts is the first step toward explaining it, especially with a subject so complicated as the mind.

5-3 (b) Splitting the mind.

Thus, our daily experience fits neatly with Chalmers' notion of two separate aspects to the mind, or even two separate minds. One is the realm of conscious experience, which is vivid, private and incommunicable. The other is the realm of knowledge and decisions, which is silent, public and communicable. The brain has two distinct functional aspects, as follows:

DUAL ASPECT THEORY OF MIND	
Mind as **CONSCIOUS EXPERIENCE**	Mind as **KNOWLEDGE FUNCTIONS**
PRIVATE	PUBLIC
VIVID	SILENT
INCOMMUNICABLE	COMMUNICABLE

Fig. 5-1: The Dual Aspect Theory of Mind

There are many examples of a single entity acquitting two functions: consider the endocrine and the exocrine functions of the pancreas, or a car, which can be both a means of transport and a status symbol, or even a central bank, which has to supply banknotes as well as guarantee price stability. This everyday fact relies on the concept of "multiple realizability," the idea that function occupies a different realm of discourse from structure. A single function can arise through different structures, and a single structure can have different functions. Daily experience shows that the brain gives rise to two very different mental functions; our task is to make sense of this. However, if the brain generates two functionally separate minds, we need to have some explanation of this peculiar fact as well as showing how they interact.

To show how this is done, consider a simple experiment. A subject is seated in a comfortable chair in a completely dark, silent room. His eyes are open and fixed somewhere in front of him. The experiment consists of a small, brief flash of green light directly in front of his field of vision. When he sees it, he must say aloud what has happened. As soon as he has said the word *green,* or *vert,* or *hijau,* he stands up, collects his money and leaves. That's all. Now what has happened to him? Almost as soon as the light flashes on, he becomes aware of something small and round and green in front of him, where previously there was just darkness. At the same time, he becomes aware of the knowledge concept, *greenness,* which immediately translates into one of the various words for greenness in the world's languages. That is, a single event in the physical world gives rise, almost simultaneously, to two very different mental events, one in the realm of conscious experience and one in the realm of knowledge functions. However, our subject has used only one sensory receptor, so the two mental events must have arisen somehow from a single data input.

If we follow the path of the sensory input, we can see that the stimulus causes only certain of the retinal receptors to fire; this leads to a barrage of impulses in the optic nerve which can readily be traced back to the brainstem, and thence via the optic radiation to the striate cortex. Unfortunately, once in the cortex, the pattern becomes too complex for current technology to follow but, very soon after, the subject will report his experience. Somewhere, almost certainly in the association cortex, the impulses are split, with some of the informational flow evoking his private conscious experience of *greenness* and some generating the public knowledge function manifest as him saying "It's green." The first response is to assume that there are two separate dedicated neuronal circuits involved because, ordinarily, activity in a single pathway would result in only a single outcome. However, there may be another, more economical explanation for the two realms, which I will outline later.

We need to explain these two realms, the experiential and the cognitive, translating the mentalist phenomena in the list at the beginning of this section, into simplified mechanisms based in biological functions, but it isn't that easy. With conscious experience, we haven't a clue where to start. Chalmers called this the really difficult bit of any theory of mind, but he insisted we could not dismiss it. However, we can put it aside for the time being because, when it comes to explaining rapid, silent knowledge functions, we are on much stronger ground.

5-4. Turing's Account of Mindless Mentation

5-4 (a) Calculators don't need homunculi

The usual understanding of the mind is that, somewhere in the head, there is a hidden person (or Soul, ego, Self or I) who surveys the sensory input then quickly scans the memory banks to reach a decision. This approach, similar to Descartes' model of substance dualism or the spiritual Self in Popper and Eccles [4], is not an explanation at all. All it does is shift that which requires explanation one dimension away from the realm of observation, meaning it starts an infinite regress and is therefore non-scientific. It also generates a further, intractable problem, of how information gets from one realm to the other, the well-known Mind-Body problem. In order to explain mentation, we must begin the process of decomposing cognitive function into its basic elements, so that we can give an explanation of recognizing a face without invoking a person doing the recognizing. That is, we have to give an account of mental functions in terms which do not presume the question to be answered, meaning we require a natural materialist (non-conscious) account of knowledge functions.

Fortunately, we have very many materialist models of non-conscious decision-making, ranging from sea-slugs to children's toys, from computers to human reflexes. Despite their variety, all of these models rely on the principles worked out in 1936 by a British mathematician, Alan Turing [5, 6]. While Turing knew little about biology, the principles he established are fundamental to our understanding of the control of behavior. Note that I have moved from talking about mental life to the notion of control, mainly because I think terms such as consciousness or mentality are hopelessly misleading. If we ask how humans are controlled, we get a much more sensible answer than if we ask, "What is the nature of consciousness?"

My case is that humans are controlled by mental events, but not as we ordinarily use the term. People look for the controlling locus in human affairs in the brilliant, sparkling realm of conscious experience, that familiar circus in the head which almost never takes a break. In fact, the locus of control lies in the silent and greatly underestimated realm of cognitive functions. Freud talked of "unconscious decisions" but all decisions are, in any practical sense of the word, unconscious, just because cognitive functions are not in the realm of conscious experience. They are beyond introspection just because they are profoundly different in nature, separate from and never part of conscious experience. We do not know how we know something, all we know is that we know it. I can recognize a human face, and immediately decide if I have seen it before. However, I don't know how I recognize a face from a lemon because any explanation I offer will always bog down in brute facts: I can only say: "Well, it looks like a face." In fact, my brain tells me if I have seen a face before, it isn't something I work out for myself. How do I know that the conscious human mind isn't involved in these decisions? Because chimps and babies are just as good at it as I am. I glance around and, yes, that face is familiar but that one is not but, very often, animals are better at these decisions than we are. Whatever process works for humans is almost certainly working for animals, too.

In the abstract realm, I know injustice when I see it but I don't know how I know it. If I write a poem, I don't know where the rhymes come from, all I do is select the best one. These are unconscious functions in every sense of the word. That is, cognitive or knowledge functions take place very rapidly without anything approximating a deliberate, willed input. Can we assemble a model of unconscious decision-making? I believe that, using the concepts developed by Turing, we can elaborate a model of human cognitive function which gives a natural (non-magical) account of how our subject can know that what he saw was green. This leads to a model of behavior, including emotion, and thence to a model of mental disorder.

5-4 (b) Mindless calculation in the brain

Turing was interested in the principles underlying any calculating machine. He showed that if the steps in any computation are reduced to the level at which a machine had only to respond with yes or no to a lengthy series of questions, then any practical calculation could be performed by a machine. The mechanism he proposed was devastatingly simple: an input tape, a memory, a read/write head, a control or checking function and an output tape [Fig. 5-2].

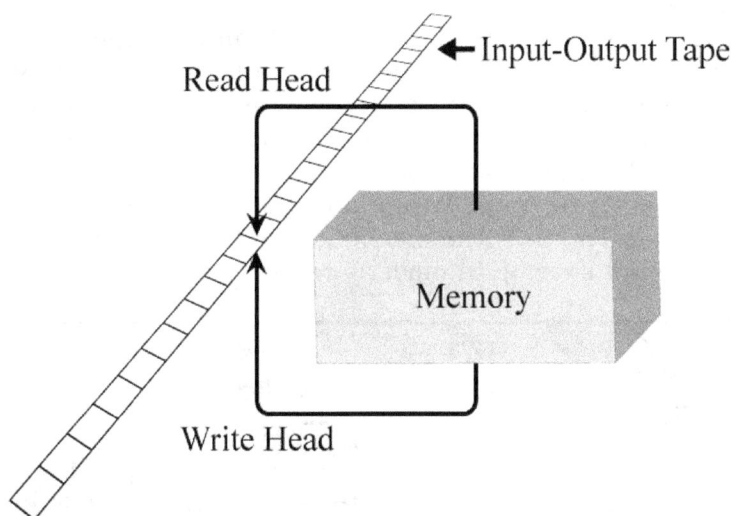

Fig. 5-2: Elements of a Turing Machine

The input tape is simplified to the point of inanity, such that the data can be in one of only two forms, a one or a zero. All the machine has to do is read each datum sequentially, compare it with its memory store and decide whether to leave it as it is, or change it. Crucially, this is all machine-based: there is no thought in it whatsoever. This is exactly how sea slugs function at the neuronal level. In fact, it doesn't even need to be electrical or chemical. The original computer was Charles Babbage's Analytical Engine, the first design of which dated from 1837. It was purely mechanical, yet it could undertake surprisingly high levels of computation. Blaise Pascal had designed one in 1642 but probably never made it.

In Turing's model, the output data flow is in the same form as the input data because nothing has transformed it. Similarly, the memory has to be in the same form otherwise it can't be compared. This simple model is called a discrete state machine. It can perform only a single function because the memory is fixed, and can be in only one of two states with nothing in between. However, Turing showed that, by coding the instructions in the input tape itself, a machine with a sufficiently large memory could perform an infinite number of functions. The machine can only respond to the state of the tape but, if instructions are coded into the tape, it will change its function accordingly. He named this the universal computing machine but we know it as the Turing machine. The significant feature is that all calculations take place in a single realm. There is no jump or transition from matter to ectoplasm, and this is exactly what we need to account for Chalmers' psychological or cognitive realm. As long as all the input tracts, the memory, all instructions and the output tracts are in a single form, then we potentially have a materialist model of all human knowledge functions, meaning a theory to account for half of our mental function. By keeping information processing out of the conscious realm, we sidestep the dualist's nightmare, the problem of how to get information in and out of the conscious realm. What I know, and what I see, are two different things and as long as they don't interact, no ontological injustice is done.

Of course, one clunky tape-reading machine isn't going to account for the speed and complexity of human decisions. We are very good at making decisions, because our survival depends on it. Over hundreds of millions of years, evolutionary pressures have selected for a high speed and accurate multimodal decision-maker, which is essentially how we function. If we connect an array of single Turing processors, then their functional diagram will be akin to Fig. 5-2. The machines send data to each other and back to themselves (not shown). In modern parlance, they "talk" to each other.

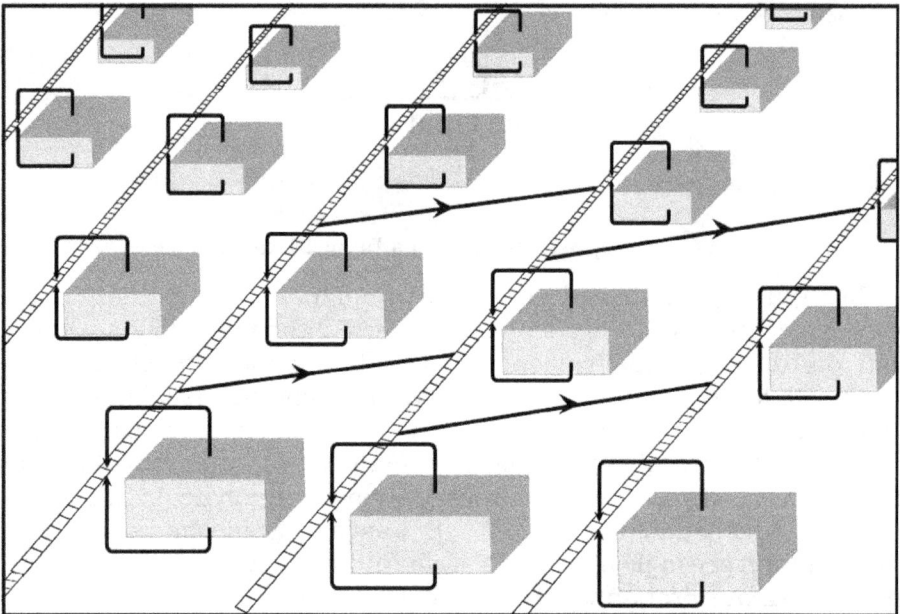

Fig. 5-2: An array of Turing machines in three dimensions.

Unfortunately, it is impossible to represent the complexity of the three-dimensional interconnections on paper but, on first principles, anything arranged in this manner would have prodigious computing capacity. There are striking similarities between this stylized picture, and the functional computational module or column of the cerebral cortex, as detailed by

Mountcastle in his historic paper [7]. As presently understood, neurons are clustered in functional groups oriented perpendicular to the cortical surface. The basic element is the cortical minicolumn of about 25μm across; 80-100 of these are grouped into the typical cortical column or module, which is about 600μm across and 3mm deep. Several dozen columns form a local cortical area network, which is the functional cortical unit or module [8]. Since there are about two million cortical modules joined together in ways we have not yet imagined, I suggest this gives the physical and mathematical basis of a biological computing machine whose limits we haven't reached. Indeed, it might, in principle, be capable of computing any possible problem in the universe. I do not believe this is an outlandish claim. Based on simple, repetitive units, the adaptive immune system is almost certainly capable of recognizing and responding to any possible organic compound from anywhere in the universe [9], and the brain is very, very much more complex than the immune system.

5-4 (c). Hidden homunculi

There are three immediate objections to this notion. First, Turing's universal computing machine was conceived as an assembly of metal and glass and paper; in order to utilize it, we have to show that it can be instantiated in biological form. In fact, this is easy. Turing wasn't at all interested in how the machine would be put together, his only interest lay in what it did. Accordingly, as long as a machine can perform the broad tasks he set, it can function as a universal computer. That means it can be in biological form. Secondly, there is certainly nothing in biology that can equate with a moving tape, which seems to be central to his idea. Once again, we can overcome that objection fairly easily. All we need is a model of a variable input being compared with a fixed memory, because that is all his model does. His input data arrived by paper, while ours all arrive electronically. It's just a matter of economy. In biology, we certainly have a huge range of examples which satisfy this requirement.

Finally, and most significantly, what does it mean to say that a machine "reads" an input, "compares" it with a memory and then "decides" what to do with it? In Turing's words, the executive unit "...carries out the various individual operations involved in a calculation" while the control ensures "that these instructions are obeyed correctly and in the right order" [4]. As it stands, isn't this just a cheap magician's trick, a homunculus or "little man" hidden inside the head? It must not be forgotten that the formal objection to homunculi is not, as Dennett supposed, that they necessarily imply substance dualism, or ectoplasm, as he scathingly termed it, but because they set up an infinite regress. So in order for Turing's model to be convincing in human psychology, we need to be able to render these processes in physical form, to show a real mechanism that can actualize the conceptual steps involved in reading, comparing and calculating. In fact, we have good conceptual and practical examples of machines reading and comparing and deciding right from wrong, devices that work so well that we trust our lives to them. The central functional elements in these machines are called logic gates, and this model of mind depends utterly on them. If we didn't have logic gates to actualize the processes of intellect, then my alleged model would be no better than the smoke and mirrors of the psychoanalysts or of crude biological claims. My suggestion is that the logic gate is the point of contact between the insubstantial world of mind and the solid world of physics and biology. Everything that passes from one world to the other must go, as it were, through a "logic gate."

5-5. Conclusion

Traditional models of mind failed to distinguish between the different mental subfunctions, meaning theorists were trying to find a single explanation to account for a diverse range of mental phenomena. Classically, the mental functions were assigned to a spirit or, as we would now say, a homunculus. This is not a scientific explanation as it merely begins an infinite regress, but it also institutionalizes another problem, of how information jumped the gap from body to mind and back again, without violating any fundamental physical laws. Over time, the concept of physical-mental interaction has been so intractable that many have despaired of ever resolving the "mind-body problem."

Over the past century, there have been several novel attempts to eliminate the mentalist element in explanations of human behavior. For psychiatry, the most significant were behaviorism, which denied any causative role for mental life, and reductionist biologism, which says that mentality can be reduced directly to the physical brain with no loss of explanatory power. These accounts have manifestly failed, meaning psychiatry is left without a working model of mind to use as the basis for its concept of mental disorder. In fact, there cannot be a non-mentalist account of human behavior.

However, approaching the phenomena of mental life from a different direction allows us to begin the process of giving a rational account of this "world knot." By splitting the whole of mental life into two distinct parts, we can readily derive an explanation for the knowledge functions based in well-recognized principles developed in other fields of science. This eliminates the conceptual homunculus which has bedeviled dualist models of mind throughout history, not because of substance dualism but because of the concealed infinite regress. However, the principles have to be translated into biological reality, and this requires three further conceptual steps.

6 Embodied Logic

"Facts which at first seem improbable will, even on scant explanation, drop the cloak which has hidden them and stand forth in naked and simple beauty."
Galileo Galilei, from Dialogues Concerning Two New Sciences *(1638).*

6-1. Introduction

In Chapter 5, it was suggested we should regard the knowledge-based functions of the mind as similar in principle to the functions of any machine which operates in the computational realm. The theoretical basis of automated decision-making is that any question can be broken down into a sequence of sub-decisions. In turn, each of these can be further reduced to a long series of elemental questions of such simplicity that a machine can answer them simply by following rules. The separate decisions are then reassembled until, eventually, the answer to the original question emerges. An observer who has not been aware of the mechanical processes between question and answer may attribute the decision to some sort of magic but there is nothing magic about the process. Decisions only seem to be intelligent if we don't realize the complexity of the automated processes between question and answer. If we can show that intelligence isn't really that smart after all, then we are well on the way to a non-question-begging, materialist theory of mind, the *sine qua non* of a scientific theory of dualist interaction.

However, it is one thing to announce: "Here is the principal by which the brain makes its myriad daily decisions," but it is another thing altogether to have a mechanism by which that principle is realized. In order to progress toward the goal of a materialist theory of mind, we need something to turn theory into practicality. We need to relate the generic principle Turing elaborated in his universal computing machine to a specific brain mechanism which, ideally, we can see under a microscope. That is, we need to find a high-speed manipulator of stupendously large data flows which is capable of functioning at unimaginable levels of accuracy year in, year out, such that the human species can survive and prosper in a harsh environment. We now have not just the generic principle, but also the precise theoretical mechanism and, crucially, a brain process that can acquit that mechanism. Granted, this is a bold claim so I will take some time to justify it.

6-2. The Brain as a Logic Machine

6-2 (a) Innate logical operations

At the time Turing was conducting his theoretical research, in the mid-1930s, there was nothing like a computing machine in existence. The word computer meant the people, mostly young ladies, who laboriously performed the columns of calculations mathematicians used in their research. The computers, being the ladies who computed, were required to adhere to precisely defined formulae with no room for imagination. Turing wanted to replace them with an infallible machine that worked at blinding speed and never needed to powder its nose. As a diversion, he began building a computing machine from scratch but he worked alone and others were beginning to race ahead. His theoretical work was interrupted by the Second World War, which took him further into practical applications of mathematics, and only much later was he involved in building the first British computer. However, the crucial mechanisms for translating his theory into a working machine had been described years before.

Computation depends on rules, specifically the rules of logic, and those rules have to be put into a physical form or embodied before the computing machine can take shape. The rules of logic are precisely-defined relationships, and one thing that machines do very well is operate according to defined relationships. They adhere to precisely-defined relationships with no variation, just because they are built to do nothing else (except break down). Machines are controlled by the laws of the physical universe, especially the laws of thermodynamics. What a computing machine does is co-opt those laws to the realm of logical relationships. In a biological sense, it is akin to the way viral particles co-opt the machinery of the host cell, giving it new instructions so that the cell does their reproductive work for them. The rules of logic cannot breach any of the rules of the physical universe but they can transcend them temporarily by expending energy. By this means, they can drive a process in a direction the laws of thermodynamics would not normally permit.

Pre-war, when Turing was doing his original work, the relationships defined by physical machines were relationships between physical things, like steel cogs, fluid pressures or electric charges, and they therefore existed only in the physical world. However, even though the rules of logic define precise relationships, they are not of a physical form. Therefore, to build a logic machine, he needed a mechanism for manipulating inputs. Since he knew the rules of logic, meaning the relationships between input and output, all he had to do was find a device that duplicated those relationships in physical form. The search was greatly simplified by the fact that the input states or signals of formal logic are restricted to units, otherwise the rules of valid inference become impossibly complex. The physical form which embodies the computational rules is now known as a logic gate, or logic gates, as there are quite a number of them. By co-opting the laws of the physical universe, logic gates embody or actualize the notion of truth (and thereby falsity), and are therefore the most basic working elements of any machine that can manipulate truth and falsity. Truth and falsity, of course, are the basis for all decisions, and decisions are the basis of all intelligent behavior.

At this point, we need to define the term 'logic' because it is fundamental to the case being developed. There are various definitions, but the two I prefer are:

> Logic is the study of valid inference; or
> Logic is the study of consistent sets of beliefs.

A set of beliefs is consistent if there is some possible situation by which they could all be true. A set is inconsistent if there is no possible situation by which they could be true, i.e. they are self-contradictory. Regardless of the definition, logic studies non-physical or contextual relationships which we grasp intuitively (i.e. without education). If we look at physical objects, such as wooden blocks, it is clear that there can be many physical relationships, such as 'on top of,' 'beside,' 'larger than,' 'faster than,' and so on. Even though we describe them in terms of a reference system, such as the standard Newtonian physics, we aren't much better at discerning or manipulating these physical relationships than chimps. The development of this form of cognitive function in humans was first explored by Jean Piaget and has since been studied in great detail in humans and many other animals. We are born with it, it is practically the same in all higher-order primates [1], it gives us vital information about the world and, without it, we wouldn't be here today. However, when we talk about cognitive functions as logical operations, we mean more than just this simple type of cognition. Using the analogy of the immune system, which has two subsystems, the innate and the adaptive, I want to distinguish clearly between two parts of the cognitive system, which can also be called the innate and the adaptive systems. The innate cognitive system (ICS), which is probably common to all higher primates, does not undertake logical processes as we normally use the term, they are reserved to the adaptive cognitive system (ACS).

There is now a very large if rather disorganized literature on the ICS of a wide range of animals. It is, however, of crucial importance not to confuse the ICS with what people like to call consciousness. With innate cognition, we are talking about decision-making which is both high-speed and silent, meaning not open to introspection. Innate cognition is the primary basis for behavioral control in all animals. It has nothing to do with what people usually mean when they say "mind," i.e. languages and symbols, or the experience of colors and odors. It has to do with alarm among baboons if they see something slithering through the grass toward them, or young children panicking if they can't see the face of a parent in the room, or recoiling from frogs but reaching out to stroke a kitten. It is concerned with what we call body-language, with threat and affection displays, of how a crying baby cannot be ignored, of pheromones and sexual arousal, defeat and sexual inhibition, of how puppies attract while maggots repel, or how the scent of roses soothes while the odor of putrefaction nauseates. It is about dominance, xenophobia, territoriality, greed and possessiveness, the darker side of human life, or what some people call human nature.

To be precise, because it is also about chimp and baboon life, we should refer to the innate cognitive system as higher primate nature. It is a crude and primitive system, mediated by the visceral brain and driven by emotions as the propulsive force. This is a huge, genetically-determined, reservoir of unthinking behavioral responses directed at surviving in a dangerous world—actually, the particular dangerous world in Africa several million years ago. There is still debate over its exact mechanism, and I will return to this point. I should emphasize that "unthinking" does not mean "reflex" as the behaviorists used it. A lot of people would like to think the ICS doesn't exist, that we are born *tabula rasa* or have somehow outgrown it ("halfway between angels and animals"), but it is a fact and if we ignore it for ideological reasons, we do so at our peril.

6-2 (b) Acquired logical operations

Humans, however, have a further system of survival. We don't survive by our senses because, apart from our color vision, they really aren't very good. Thus, a young bear sees two mountain lions go into its cave but only one comes out. The bear doesn't go in, not because it can count but because it can still smell the other predator. We can't do that, our sense of smell isn't good enough, but we can tell the difference between one and two. Very early, children realize that if they put a toy in the cupboard, it should still be there when they go back. Soon, they realize they can hide things, and then tell lies about it. These are Piaget's cognitive operations and they represent the fundamental basis of our formal systems of logic. Logic is nothing more than valid inference about relationships in the material world. It says things like, "If you have two apples and you eat one, there won't be two next time you look." It says, "You can't be in two places at the same time," that everything has a cause and, "What goes up must come down." If it is true that dogs are scent detectors, rabbits are sound detectors and birds are movement detectors, then humans are relationship detectors. That's how we survive, just because we don't smell or hear or see as well as other animals we might want to eat or that might want to eat us.

It must be understood that these types of logical relationships are of the natural world; this does not apply to what is usually called the supernatural world. Indeed, the main purpose of invoking a supernatural world is to explain the gaps in our rational understanding of the natural world. But as our knowledge of relationships of the universe expands, so religion shrinks, until all it can claim is the one thing for which we have no evidence, what (if anything) happens after death. The supernatural is about irrationality, but rationality is the basis of the adaptive cognitive system. We can see its survival value, we can understand the theoretical basis for it, and we can see that the brain actually has the computing power to manage it, but what is the precise mechanism? If a chimp and a human look at the same object, how can the human's visual input be transposed into abstract logical systems? The answer is by logic gates, which doesn't mean as much as it sounds. One professor defined logic gates as devices which process one or more input signals in a logical fashion, which is not very helpful.

A logic gate is any ordered physical system or device which performs regular operations upon or manipulates input signals, such that the relationship between input and output signals varies regularly, and exactly parallels in physical form one of more of the relationships defined by the rules of formal logic. The interest here lies in the way input and output activity can be equated with the concept of truth. The simplest logical relationship is the unary operator, *Not* (negation). By definition, this operates on a single input, and converts it to its opposite. In electronics, the unary operator is usually known as an inverter. If the input is positive, the output is negative, and vice versa. There doesn't appear to be a limit to the nature of the physical machines that can function as unary operators: they can be physical, chemical or electronic. Even a door is a logic gate (enter vs. not enter). Remember that gates can be connected in series, one after the other, so that the output of one gate becomes the input of another gate, or a gate's output may act back upon its own input or upon its own function. Feedback and feed forward loops open the possibility of converting a controlled function to a self-controlled function.

Binary operators act upon two input signals to produce a single output in a relationship which precisely and predictably parallels the logical relationships that exist between two entities in the abstract realm. The simplest binary operator is addition, where one apple and another apple equals two apples. Similarly, subtraction is absolutely elementary to our understanding of the world: two cats go in, one comes out, means one is still hanging around inside. A bucket with a small hole in it is a simple example of a logic gate. It says:

"Liquids will escape, leaving the solids behind."

In formal notation, we can represent this sentence as follows:

$$[(\text{Liquid} \rightarrow \text{Escape}) \wedge (\text{Solid} \rightarrow \neg \text{Escape})].$$

The simple mechanism of a hole in a bucket exactly parallels what we intuitively understand of relationships in the real world. Assuming we have the capacity to distinguish solids and liquids, which is not a bad assumption because chimps and infants can, then all we need is a mechanism for recognizing specific relationships, such as negation, conjunction, material implication, etc. in order to develop an abstract realm (Note that I did not say "in order to *enter* an abstract realm," because, in the materialist ontology, it isn't "up there" waiting for us as it doesn't exist until we develop it). I believe such a mechanism does exist, but it is simplicity itself because it is nothing more than a tiny modification of normal neuronal function.

Look at another example:

"When the starting pistol fires, you should run until the checkered flag falls."

In logic, it would read:

$$[(\text{Bang} \rightarrow \text{Run}) \wedge (\text{Flagfall} \rightarrow \text{Stop})].$$

In physiological terms, we would translate this as:

"Activity in the acoustic detector activates the leg mover until it is terminated by a visual input."

Without much effort, we can train chimps to do this but only humans can do it simply from reading the directions. There is an exact parallel between the physical system of the brain and the abstract system of a foot race. However, this is a simple example, what about a difficult one? The same principles hold, embodied in the same mechanisms, but with a specific elaboration.

The basic *AND* logic gate is built in such a way that not all outputs are possible. An *AND* gate is any mechanism which has two inputs, *A* and *B*, but only allows an output *C* when both inputs are active. All other combinations are forbidden. An *OR* gate allows an output *C* when either *A* or *B* is activated, or both, but will remain inactive when neither *A* nor *B* is active. There are many possible variations and formats [2]. If, however, we designate an active input as *Truth*, and the inactive state as *Falsity*, then it will change from being a processor of apples or footraces into a processor of truth and falsity. That is, it will form the basis of all abstract thought, meaning a cognitive system which can adapt to the world. It is in this crucial respect, an adaptive cognitive system, that allows *H. sapiens* to dominate the world, not baboons.

Fig. 6-1 illustrates the notion of "mindless decision-making." The shape of a circle is recognized at the lower levels of retina and mid-brain; this is a simple matter of on-off detectors firing in a particular pattern. Artificial models of circle-recognition are easy to devise. Similarly, the color red is recognized at the retinal level: there is no intervention of anything like a "conscious level" of choice. Thus, the brain is capable of detecting a red circle without our "human features" intervening. Chimps and birds can do this with ease. If this aptitude is then combined with a human memory ("If red circle, then press foot"), which also interacts at a neuronal level, then we have a model of non-conscious decision-making. This does not imply that there is no intent: with qualification, I choose what rules I will commit to memory, the qualification being that I can extract rules (as generalizations) from my environment with forming a fully-conscious intent to do so. But they are always my rules: I have the capacity to become aware of my rules, even if I don't know how they work. A person can learn that his accent is not chic, even if he has no knowledge of when he learned it or how he manages to speak without, say, enunciating consonants (for example, when some people say the word *Federal*, it sounds like *feral*, which is perhaps not inappropriate). So this model, which relies heavily on the notion of non-conscious decision-making, provides no escape for the criminal who claims: "I don't know, your Honor, I just found myself breaking into the store and running off with the till." In theory and in fact, we are responsible for our decisions.

To summarize, just as immunology has two closely-related systems, the innate and the adaptive immune systems, so too cognitive psychology has two closely-related systems, one innate and one adaptive. The innate cognitive system is a relatively simple matter of the crude processing of data arriving from exteroceptors in simple neuronal systems which are directly connected to effector organs. Effector organs include not only hands, feet and mouths, but also the genitalia, the larynx and, critically for psychiatry, the organs of emotion, whatever they are. 350 years ago, Descartes said that the body is just a machine. He was absolutely right: all that separates the sensory receptors and the effector organs is a bit of mindless data-crunching. For example, the retina detects certain patterns in the visual environment, conveys its information to the striate cortex which computes a response and sends instructions to the feet. Birds do it, bees do it, and even children's toys do it.

But by interposing a new array of slightly-modified neurons between the receptors and the effectors, the human brain gains a modified or adaptive cognitive system which is vastly more effective in detecting and computing relationships in the real world. The modified neurons function as truth and falsity processors or logic gates, but we usually know them by the collective term, association cortex. Of course, all primates have association cortex, but ours is very much bigger, thereby giving us an edge over chimps. If the output of a level of logic gates then becomes the input of the next level, so that logical output is processed and reprocessed, then the permutations of the final output are magnified exponentially. That is, simply by the interposition of perhaps half a dozen layers of modified neurons between input and output, the human behavioral repertoire becomes many millions of times more complex than that of our nearest relatives. Animals have logic gates, of course: primary receptors and primary cortex work by essentially the same principles, and human receptors and primary cortex are substantially the same as those seen in chimps. However, their first-order data processing or innate cognitive system is directed to the effector organs whereas ours is reprocessed in the association cortex before being routed to the final effector organs.

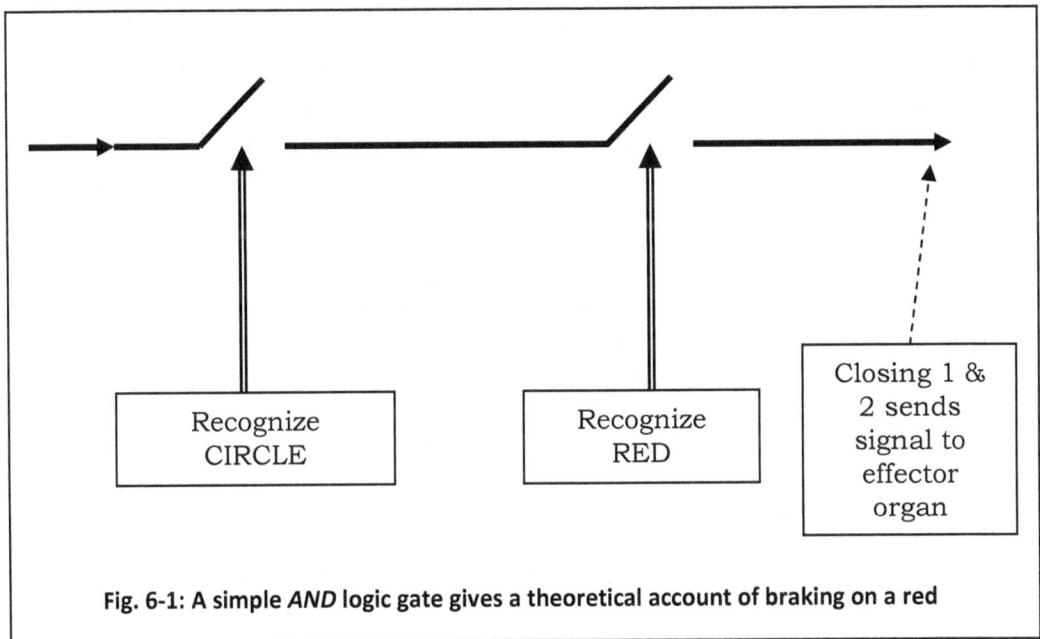

Fig. 6-1: A simple *AND* logic gate gives a theoretical account of braking on a red

So we can now answer Kandel's claim that bird calls and human language should be amenable to the same biological analysis [4, p400]: this is most definitely not true. The secondary or higher order logic gates, which humans alone have, allow us to dissimulate, and there is no biological analysis that will allow us to differentiate between truth and falsity, just because they are not biological constructs. In evolutionary terms, it may be that the biggest advantage wrought by the adaptive cognitive system is that it gives us the capacity for deception.

6-3. The Mechanism of the Brain's Logic Gates

It is all very well to claim: "Here is a mechanism for rendering abstract notions such as truth and falsity in physical form, but the most important step is to prove that this actually happens in the brain. Unless we can find an exact biological mechanism as the substrate for logical processes, the model being developed in this book will not succeed. Fortunately, recent advances in neurophysiology indicate that not only do such mechanisms exist, but they function exactly as required by the model.

The essential feature of any logic gate is that it permits the manipulation of inputs in a stereotyped way, leading to a restricted range of outputs. Among the body's many different cell types, only neurons seem to have the requisite features: very fast acceptance, manipulation and transfer of inputs which leave little or no trace of their passage. Furthermore, nerve endings function as transducers, detecting specific energy inputs from the environment and translating them into high speed data flows in the nervous system which can be further processed and manipulated as they travel through the system. Thus, we have an input side, in which sensory organs collect information from the environment, transducing it and then transferring it to the central processsing site before it is directed to specific effector organs. In essence, this is no different from the carefully detailed models of animal neural control assembled by generations of minutely detailed work by researchers, from Ramon y Cajal, to Hodgkin and Huxley, to Eccles, Hubel and Weisel, Kandel and so many others. Many of these historic characters have been honored by the Nobel Prize and rightly so. They have changed our entire understanding of the biological world. However, the crucial question is whether their work has any application to psychiatry. Can the ordinary principles of neuronal transmission be co-opted to the processing of truth and falsity?

Basic neural physiology is covered in any standard text [4, 5, 6]. Neurons are excitable cells due to their unstable cell membranes, and interneural transmission is electrochemical in nature. All information in the brain is in the form of coded neural impulses travelling from one nerve to the next, effected by a large (and growing) range of neurotransmitters, the chemicals which bridge the gaps between individual neurons. Neurotransmitters can be either excitatory or inhibitory, and can have short or long term effects. The classic short-term effect is seen at the synapse, where an impulse releases chemicals into the synaptic cleft, allowing them to diffuse across the cleft and alter the membrane potential in the post-synaptic neuron. This is very fast, with the chemicals being released and deactivated or reabsorbed into the presynaptic nerve terminal in the order of milliseconds.

If we look at the peripheral sensory receptors, such as the retina, we understand fairly well how the eye generates a very accurate, real-time image of the world around us [7]. The retina functions at high speeds by principles which remain strictly within the realm of materialist science. There is nothing mysterious about the mechanism of sight, or of hearing or sensation. Moving into the CNS proper, nerves conduct according to the principles discovered eighty years ago by Huxley and Hodgkin using squid neurons. Similarly, the output state of the brain consists of cascades of nervous impulses in dedicated systems which control the activity of a huge range of somatic and visceral organs. What happens between input and output involves no magic. That is, action potentials of CNS neurons are no different from those in peripheral nerves, either afferent or efferent, but they can achieve more than the mere conduction of information, because the neuronal cell bodies can be rapidly influenced by different inputs, to the point where they can manipulate their own output with a barely measurable delay. That is, the "ordered physical system (of the neuron) performs regular operations upon or manipulates input signals, thereby varying the output signals such that the relationship between input and output exactly parallels in physical form one or more of the relationships defined by the rules of formal logic." Because their physical structure allows them to switch rapidly from one state to another, the normal function of clusters of neurons is co-opted to function as "processors of truth and falsity... (thereby forming)... the basis of all abstract thought, meaning a cognitive system which can adapt to the world."

This broad principle needs qualification. Firstly, not all manipulation of the data flow takes place at the axo-dendritic junction [8]. Cerebral neurons have huge numbers of terminals on the cell body, as many as 10,000 per soma, all of which influence whether the cell fires an impulse or not. There are many known neurotransmitters, probably eighty or more, and each of these can be either excitatory or inhibitory. Post-synaptic potentials summate according to a Boolean process, meaning our present understanding of neuronal function meets the essential criteria of logic gates. Secondly, the input to the CNS is in the form of data flows coded into neuronal impulses, and the output of the CNS is in exactly the same form. As previously described [9], the most parsimonious explanation of what happens between input and output is that it should remain in the same form in the physical realm. That is, so long as the information remains in the form of data coded into neuronal impulses, and does not leave the material realm, there is no need for a homunculus such as the soul to make the decisions that distinguish humans from chimps. Automated decisions are a fact of chimp life: not only is there no *a priori* reason for the human brain to be different, but there is also clear evidence that critical parts of the human and *Pan* brains use the same codes to perform the same task [1]. However, because it has complex arrays of neurons functioning at different levels of complexity between input and output, the human brain can make vastly more complicated decisions than a chimp brain. This will not convince everybody: as Turing himself noted some sixty years ago, there are plenty of people who will never believe that machines can do what humans do. They insist that humans have something extra that monkeys and machines can never have. He believed his opponents would never allow themselves to be convinced otherwise: as soon as somebody shows that a machine can do what they said was impossible, they will move the target [10].

This raises a critically important point. If the brain functions (at least in part) as a digital data processor which, every minute of the day, generates the myriad decisions we need to stay alive, does this 1300gm organ have enough raw computing power? It has been suggested that only quantum computing could account for the complexity of human behavior and experience [11]. My suggestion is that we do not need to invoke the unfathomable to explain our behavior, that the human brain uses the same processing principles as other species [12] and does in fact have sufficient power to explain behavior:

> "A principal result from the vast majority of imaging studies is that every cognitive process is supported by a widespread constellation of activated areas extending throughout the brain. Although this conclusion may often be obfuscated by the drastic restriction in field of view that ensues from excessive significance thresholding or region-of interest selection, functional neuroimaging results generally support the existence of distributed neurocognitive networks in the brain... When examined from this perspective, cognition is seen as a dynamic process that rapidly evolves through a series of informationally consistent coordination states. In each moment of cognitive processing, the cognitive microstate is defined by the selective coordination of local cortical area networks that are interacting by virtue of their interconnectivity within the large scale anatomical structure of the cortex (p143-4).

A very large part of human mental activity can be seen in other animals, so no special processes need be invoked to account for them. For the rest, it is important to recall that each neuron is not just a single logic gate, it is a microprocessor in its own right. Each neuronal cell body receives as many as 10,000 inputs and synapses with perhaps a further 2,000 neurons. Bearing in mind the large numbers of known neurotransmitters, that means each cell body probably has many hundreds of logic gates, integrating data from a variety of sources and transmitting it forward to perhaps thousands of destinations. There are something like 2,000,000 cortical module, each of which has in the order of 10,000 neurons, and if every neuron in each module receives an average of 5,000 inputs giving rise to several hundred logic gates, it is clear that the data-processing capacity of the human brain is enormous (see Fig. 6-2). Furthermore, the arrays of neural processors are in parallel, not in series, which greatly magnifies the channel capacity of the brain. With distributed parallel processing of data, there is almost certainly sufficient capacity in the brain to dispense with irrefutable notions, such as immortal souls or quantum processing. But this may not convince the fanatic: as with so much else that he did, Turing's pessimistic opinion on human gullibility has proved remarkably prescient.

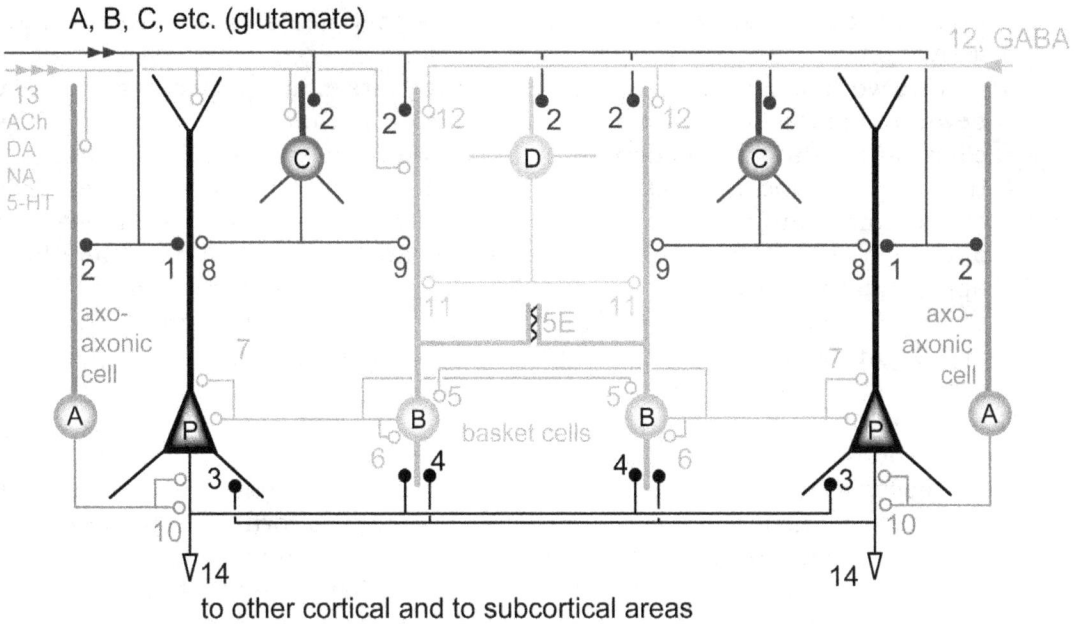

Fig. 6-2. A diagrammatic representation of cortical neuronal structure within the cortical modules.

Pyramidal cells (P) are extensively interconnected (3), as are basket cells (B, 5) which also innervate themselves through autapses (6). GABAergic cells (dark) innervate the field in a domain-specific manner. The pyramidal output (14) has extensive pre- and post-somatic inputs. This type of circuit is repeated for each of the many cerebral neurotransmitters (13) and in each of the cortical layers. The cascading pattern of data-processing gives the cortex its unique characteristic of high-speed, multichannel manipulation of information inputs to give a selective, graded output. (Modified with permission from [19]; this paper has a number of excellent diagrams and photomicrographs).

Finally, human mental function is not just a matter of current processing of sensory input. Like all animals, we don't just function in the here and now, but we learn new responses, meaning our behavior changes as a result of experience. This theory needs, therefore, a model of permanent changes in neuronal status to account for memory. Ever since Hebb first proposed that changes in synaptic strength are the physical basis of memory [13], cellular memory has been studied intensively. There is now no dispute that permanent changes occur in neurons subjected to training procedures. These can affect the soma of the neuron [8, 14], either directly or indirectly, or the synaptic region itself [15]. However, the crucial point is that permanent changes in nerves involve protein production, and protein production depends on gene activation. If there is an interruption to the mechanism of gene transcription which would normally lead to increased production of particular proteins needed to modify the synapse, then normal learning will not occur [16]. It might be that the connections between neurons are modified by permanent changes in the excitability of pre- or post-synaptic membranes, or by the growth of new synaptic junctions but, either way, specific proteins must be produced for the purpose, and this necessarily involves gene activation.

This work has been replicated over many years in many species and is now beyond dispute, but the reasonable objection is that the research involves classical conditioning experiments in invertebrates and small rodents, and there is no compelling reason to believe that all human memory is necessarily of the same nature. For example, I actually composed that sentence this afternoon while I was riding my bicycle; there was no hint of anything approximating a classical conditioning experiment. I rehearsed the words in my head, then didn't think of them again until I sat down, four hours later, and began to type them. Manifestly, internal mental events under personal control can result in lasting memory traces: I can learn things without an external stimulus, as mental life is primary, not secondary. The truly revolutionary implication here is that the normal processes of perceiving, recollecting and deciding, meaning the function of thought itself, can activate the neuron's genes to produce proteins required to form the memories the organism needs for its survival. That is, by active feedback and feed forward loops, the mind can control the brain's metabolism. Just by thinking, I can change my genes.

6-4. A Molecular Resolution of the Mind-Body Problem

There are two major features of mental function which must be given account in any explanation of mind, namely, memory and current computing capacity. Of course, on a functional level, these are intimately related as we would not be able to work out anything if we did not have a memory capacity. Physiologically, they are also closely related as each function depends on essential neuronal features which are conceptually similar, if not identical in nature.

6-4 (a). Memory as a cell-based function

It is not possible to summarize the enormous and rapidly expanding field of cell-based memory. Any textbook of neurophysiology (e.g. [4]) will give the background of this fascinating area but human memory, of course, is not understood to anything like the extent of the unfortunate laboratory rat. In the context of a theory of the functional mind, I am not concerned so much with memory as a sort of photo album of holiday snaps somewhere in the head. This blurs the focus on memory as the background knowledge we need to survive. Memory as information may well differ from memory as "pretty pictures" in the head. Without the ability to gather information on the environment, and store it immediately, humans would surely have gone the way of *Homo erectus*.

Classically, there have been two forms of memory, short and long term. In this chapter, I want to emphasize the functional role of immediate memory as the repository of a continuous stream of information extracted from the environment which is held in current awareness without actually forming part of what is commonly called the conscious mind. For example, a footballer is running down the field with the ball. From the corner of his eye, he sees a member of the opposing team closing in on him. His opponent soon falls behind and the first player can no longer see him. However, just because the second man is not visible does not mean the first man forgets him; the awareness of the other player is simply part of his knowledge state, a "knowing that" which is silent but effective. Similarly, a workman puts down one tool and picks up another. He does not forget the first tool but, without thinking about it, can reach for it when the need arises, often without even looking at it. Drivers are aware of traffic around them, parents know where their children are even when they are quiet (especially when they are quiet), I know what is behind me as I am typing, I know what that sound is even without focusing on it (crickets), I know what gear my car is in, where the cars are around me, on and on endlessly. Without this constant stream of information available for immediate use, we would simply stop functioning in any directed sense. Information comes in, it is held briefly, perhaps used, and then discarded (otherwise the brain would overload in very short order):

> "...the functional expression of a cognitive operation requires co-activation of a specific combination of interconnected local area networks. The co-activated local area networks represent a subset of the total set of possible networks in the cerebral cortex. The members of this subset act in concert as a neurocognitive network to express the cognitive operation, with each local cortical area network making its own specialized contribution... the high degree of reciprocal connectivity in the cerebral cortex mandates that every instant of sensorimotor processing involve the coordination of multiple sensory and motor areas, under guidance from executive coordinating areas such as the prefrontal cortex" [12, p143-5].

If information is coded into the brain in the manner I have suggested above, then the physical substrate of short term memory would be immediate modification of neuron excitability by chemical means, rather than physical modification of the cells themselves. An actual change in cell morphology requires time to activate the protein-building mechanism of the cell, including gene activation, and time to move the proteins into place. This takes hours to days, rather than the milliseconds required for immediate recall. There is ample evidence to suggest that short-term modification of interneuronal transmission is the actual mechanism by which information is retained in the short term. This can be effected by a variety of means, including short-term inhibition or enhancement of synaptic transmission itself, either directly or indirectly, or changes to the resting state of the pre-synaptic neuron. Longer-term changes may involve outgrowth of new synaptic junctions, or persisting changes to the resting polarization of the presynaptic neuron [17], all of which depends on gene activation. In fact, the relationship between cell changes and memory is known precisely in mollusks: "The change in the membrane potential of a key modulatory neuron is both sufficient and necessary to initiate a conditioned response in a reduced preparation and underscores its importance for associative LTM" [18]. The numbers of actual physical mechanisms involved in cell-based memory are growing rapidly and it is perfectly feasible that, like eyes, cellular substrates of memory have evolved many times.

Thus, the modern view of memory is of a two-fold function, one very short term and the other much longer in nature. Traditionally, investigation of memory proceeded by studying what were called conditioning experiments, essentially animal learning. As detailed in Chap. 2 of [9], this led to a completely erroneous view of human learning. There is no such process as "conditioning," and "conditioned reflexes" misstate the mechanisms of apprehension and retention. We would not be able to retain all the perceptual information which our senses collect for us each day so we have a rapid, erasable system which allows current input to be held for a short while and then discarded. This is mediated by rapidly reversible changes in neuronal excitability which blocks or enhances transmission. The second system also depends on changes in transmission but is much more complex. Long-term or permanent changes in cell excitability are effected by specific changes in the protein economy, which can only occur by means of the activation of the genetic material in the neuronal nucleus. Now since humans can initiate a long term memory purely by thought processes alone, without any external "unconditional stimulus," this leads inevitably to the apparently bizarre conclusion that, purely by thought processes alone, humans are able to switch on their genetic material in the process of laying down a permanent memory. I will admit that many people will have the gravest difficulty with this suggestion but it is unavoidable. If people can set up memories just by virtue of having a thought, then we are led to a new slogan: Just by thinking, I can change my genes. This is precisely the opposite of the biological approach to human mental function, which is that biology drives the brain. Not so. It is not true for humans, and probably not even true for most of what we would call higher animals.

6-4 (c). Computation as a cell-based function.

The processes by which humans make decisions are not known. Awesome technical problems stand between us and a full understanding of how we choose one path over another. We can only presume that information coded into the brain is manipulated according to the principles outlined by Alan Turing some seventy years ago. These were generic principles; they say nothing about the specifics of human cerebral function at a choice point. My suggestion, which is hardly novel, is that the cerebral cytoarchitecture acts as a manipulator of massive data flows. Current sensory input is brought to the brain by the afferent nerves in the form of neuronal action potentials. This interacts with the "standing instructions" of the individual's memory and a decision is reached. However, it should not be forgotten that this does not take much computing capacity and it is an even chance that we will never be able to identify the precise areas involved in even quite significant decisions. The real computing power is seen in the processes of putting the decision into effect.

For example, a simple decision such as standing up to go to bed involves glancing at the clock, realizing it is ten o'clock and then moving. The knowledge "Big hand on twelve, little hand on ten" involves only a tiny part of the total visual input for that brief moment; it could never be separated from the rest of the visual flow, and probably not distinguished from the total sensory input from all modalities for that split second. At the same time, there is buried somewhere in the brain a coded instruction: "If 10pm, go to bed." When this interacts with "Big hand on twelve, little hand on ten," then a vast array of information is triggered, and this is almost certainly the first and only sign of cerebral activity we will ever be able to detect. What happens is that the body is prepared for action. The heart rate and blood pressure must be changed from "seated" to "upright," a huge flow of instructions is directed to the motor system to activate relaxed muscles so that the body is lifted upright—and not propelled face forward into the opposite chair. The decision to walk occupies barely milliseconds of some tiny tract of the total neuronal computational capacity; as robotocists are well aware, the act of walking is vastly complex and involves huge afferent and efferent data flows.

This is an important principle. The major decisions on which we base our life are almost certainly no more than the briefest, phantom flickering in some part of the brain, more likely scattered around various parts of the brain in distributed mode so that we could never know what was going on. Perhaps it could be the case that the functional unit in critical decisions is as small as one cerebral cortical module which almost certainly will never be available to non-invasive investigation. It might be that the decision to go to bed involves one visual cortical module, which connects to one hippocampal memory module, and the final decision is then relayed to the prefrontal cortex for implementation. From here, instructions go to a myriad brain centers which current technology can detect, e.g. PET scanning or fMRI.

The logical conclusion to this model is that major decisions involving matters of life and death do not activate the whole brain at once. The significance of a decision is not reflected in the amount of brain tissue it involves, but in the value or weighting that the individual puts on it. This is elementary IT theory but seems to have escaped a number of influential biological psychiatrists. It is rather similar to the reaction of many famous physicians to Pasteur's discovery of bacteria: there were many great men who simply could not comprehend how anything so small and insignificant as a germ could kill a healthy man. The same could apply in psychiatry: the causation of, say, schizophrenia does not necessarily involve large tracts of nervous tissue. It could be a simple matter of a few, critically-sited units malfunctioning such that their damaging output is then spread widely throughout the whole functional brain as part of the brain's normal processes. That is not a contradictory statement.

Furthermore, there is no reason to believe that the malfunction is necessarily of an organic nature. The whole point of a complex data processor is that physical malfunctions can be mimicked by programming errors. If it is the case that the critical causative "lesion" in any mental disorder is tiny, then it is more likely to be a major programming fault affecting just a few functional elements than a widely distributed but minor physical error. If we take the brain's memory content as the totality of its programming, then this is akin to saying that schizophrenia could be the result of acquired beliefs, rules, fantasies, etc., which have a self-injurious effect on the individual. Once again, there is nothing in this claim which contradicts any known principle of cerebral function. However, there will be many great men who simply cannot comprehend how anything so fleeting and ephemeral as a thought could produce so devastating a condition as schizophrenia. My response is that global warming and all-out nuclear war are potentially devastating, and they are definitely caused by human thought, so mere madness is almost an afterthought.

6-4 (d). Memory and current computation are inseparable

In order to understand how a complex machine works, we follow the classic principle of reducing it to its physical and functional elements and seeing how they interact. This applies to computing machines just as much as it applies to physical machines; the processes by which decisions are made can be disintegrated and then reassembled, just like a fob watch. For a computational or logic machine, a decision is made when a current informational input is compared with certain standing instructions or memory, and a result computed. Decision-making is a mindless process: we have to show each and every step in the process to ensure that there are no hidden "loans on intelligence," i.e. no homunculi skulking in the peduncles.

The physical processes underlying memory and computation are very similar. They use the same cerebral machinery, otherwise these different functions could not interact. However, these functions arise from different applications of the neuronal circuitry. Memory, as detailed above, is a change in the conductive capacity of dedicated neurons. That is, the brain sets up a system of filters which channel or route the incoming information to certain restricted conclusions. This is not quite the same as Turing's idealized universal computing machine as the memory is localized while the inform-ational input moves around the brain. So in order to recognize a frog, for example, the association cortex filters the data flow in the visual pathways and directs part of it to a series of preset logic gates which are activated only when a particular stimulus is successful in passing through the gates. It is similar to a door key: we could say that the door only opens when the lock "recognizes" the key. However, this assigns mentality to the process of a key unlocking a door when what we are trying to do is remove the hidden mentality in decision-making by rendering it mechanical and non-question begging. So the fixed memory structure of the brain allows only certain signals through and, when they get through, they activate a particular memory which becomes our new knowledge state: "Aha, I see a frog." The visual input of a large grey thing with a trunk cannot get through the filters which are set to recognize frogs but will successfully trigger the knowledge state "elephant." How do we know what a frog is? That is what learning means: setting our own memory circuits as a result of experience, except humans can reset them purely by internal experience. I am not sure if any other animal can.

This process differs from the model of the digital computer which is so familiar (and so biasing). In the desk PC, instructions coded in memory are conveyed to a central processing unit where it interacts with the data input. However, humans don't have a central processing unit, otherwise known as homunculus. There is no all-knowing decision-maker hidden in the head, not in the pineal, not in the nucleus accumbens nor the prefrontal cortex. Memory just is a blind, dumb decision-maker which filters the sensory input and then triggers the activity which we experience as "recognizing a frog" or "making our minds up." But we cannot catch ourselves in the act of recognizing anything, just because it is a passive process. Our decisions are made and our minds made up for us by processes we cannot introspect. The whole point of a cognitive explanation of human function is that we have to remove the hidden mental component (that persistent and insistent little homunculus) by showing how each and every decision is the outcome of mindless processes. Until we can do that, we have not explained anything at all, we have simply set up an infinite regression by moving that which requires explanation further into the head.

6-4 (e). Meaning and mental disorder

If this model, or something like it, is correct, then it has immediate consequences for biological psychiatry. Firstly, it says that crucial decisions may involve only a tiny part of the cerebral substance, far too small to be detected by any non-invasive techniques which we either have or can imagine. The reason is that recognition is a passive process, not active. All scanning techniques are positive, they rely on activity in the target organ to tell us what is happening. But if the recognition process just is something passing through a passive filter, then we cannot tell anything about the filter itself. Secondly, the data flow to the memory segment is likely to be very small compared with the actual data input in that moment. Consider the example of a person seeing a frog on a branch some three meters away. Compared with the whole visual field at the instant the frog is seen, the frog doesn't contribute much to the total data flow in the visual tracts. For a person with a frog phobia, the few kilobytes of data contributed by a small green blob with big eyes is tiny compared with the whole Technicolor scene of trees, flowers, grass, sky, other people, the dog jumping around and so on. Add to this the data input from the ears (children squealing, radio playing, car going past, birds calling), sensation, posture, etc. and the wonder is that the brain can filter out all the unwanted noise and find the frog at all. But it does, and it does it by a series of steps that can never in principle be followed from input to reaction.

The problem for any biological model of phobias is simply this: at any time, we are filtering and correctly labeling astounding quantities of data, yet the significant input is but a miniscule part of the total data input. For the sake of argument, assume that the total data input in a ten millisecond bloc is one hundred megabytes. Our frog would comprise only a few kilobytes of that, even when visualized on the macula. Yet that tiny bit of information is sufficient to trigger a massive panic reaction in the phobic person, because the brain's memory function is set up to do just that, i.e. "small green blob with big eyes overwhelms all other current inputs and awareness as it triggers massive panic." That is what a trigger function means: a tiny action detonates a massive response. Thus, a biological analysis of brain function in a phobia will show two aspects only. Firstly, it will show activity in the visual centers but, because they are consistent, the analysis will filter them out. Secondly, there will be activity in a major area which governs the total body reaction in a panic state, but this will always appear to arise *de novo* just because the visual input filtering through the memory system will be too small to be detected. The researchers will jubilantly announce that they have discovered the "cause" of phobias, unaware that all they are seeing is the door creaking open *after* the key has been turned. Because what the biological assay (PET scan, fMRI, etc.) cannot show is the significance to the individual of the feared object. That is, the frog means danger, but bioassays cannot detect meaning just because meaning is semantic, not biological.

Meaning is hidden in the information coded into the brain at the neuronal level, and there is no biological test which can determine meaning without knowing the codes, but as soon as the test relies on the codes, it is not biological. Memories are tiny neuronal filters which passively screen incoming data for patterns just as locks passively screen all the things shoved in them until it "recognizes" the one and only one thing that has the right pattern of bumps to let the door swing open. But a lock doesn't recognize a key in any active sense of the word, it passively fails to respond until the right pattern is inserted; then it falls open. There is nothing active about it.

Continuing with phobias, all we are saying is that the person responds to a neutral stimulus in the environment as though it were a mortal threat, he is activating his fear response when objective reality says it is not necessary to save his life. As a question of physiology, there is nothing wrong with his fear response; the fact that he can experience terror shows that it is working extremely well. He is simply switching it on when there is no threat to his survival. Somewhere, somehow, he decided that the particular object was a danger to him; there is no brain pathology in making a mistake. Somewhere, a memory filter was set to activate a fear response when there was no danger. The filter is blind to what it is doing, and the frightened subject has no inner knowledge of what is happening to him because he cannot introspect this side of mental life. Decisions are made for us and we either enjoy them or suffer them, but we don't know what they are until after the mindless brain has done its work.

So if it's just a simple matter of making up my mind to change my genes (and thereby my fears and hates, my likes and dislikes), why is it so difficult? That depends on the difference between implicit and explicit learning and will be covered in the chapters on treatment. The critical message of this chapter is that, by means of specific gene activation, thought processes alone can set up the conditions which lead to changes in the brain's protein metabolism. The mind controls the brain, not vice versa.

6-5. Conclusion

We can split the totality of human mental experience (sometimes known as 'consciousness') in two quite separate parts, the vivid, public but incommunicable experiential realm and the communicable realm of silent, high-speed knowledge functions. The latter, the cognitive half, can be explained in principle using the theoretical constructs first outlined some seventy years ago by some of the century's most original and productive thinkers. Principles are interesting, but they need a mechanism before they can move off the page. In the case of models of automated decision-making, the crucial mechanism is the logic gate. A logic gate is nothing more than a simple mechanism that realizes the abstract or conceptual relationships upon which our survival depends. Recent advances in neurophysiology indicate very strongly that neurons have the capacity to function as logic gates. It seems the brain has sufficient computing power to account for a very large part of our daily activities. There is also ample evidence from different species to support the notion that memory is a cell-based property, and the indications are that human memory is no different. However, we can recall self-engendered mental events, not just external events, meaning whatever the processes of cell-based memory may be, pure thought alone can activate them. The conclusion is that, in human affairs, mental life is primary. This is a model of biological and cognitive interaction, or a bio-cognitive model of mind.

7 The Biocognitive Model

"Once stretched over a new idea, man's mind never goes back to its original dimensions."
Oliver Wendell Holmes

7-1. Introduction

The previous two chapters have outlined the case for a model of dualist interaction for psychiatry. Beginning with common observation of the phenomena of mental life, the model has been constructed in a stepwise process, showing that, if certain conditions are met, complex questions can be answered without invoking an extra entity or homunculus, i.e. without invoking magical substances or starting an infinite regress. So far, this model meets the minimal criteria for a scientific model of mind. As a result, all human cognitive functions can be explained in principle without leaving the field of materialist science. That is, we can derive a causally-effective mentalist theory that does not invoke irrefutable entities such as Self, ego and id. The model depends on a neuronal account of data processing and leads to the novel conclusion that pure mental activity (thought) can induce the genetic activity required to modify interneuronal transmission as the basis for memory functions. In this and the next few chapters, I will expand some of the concepts and show how this biocognitive model meshes with other fields of enquiry (see Fig. 7-1 on p. 103).

There are several things missing from this model of the cognitive mind. Firstly, we don't know how it runs; secondly, we don't know how it starts and, of course, it says nothing about conscious experience. But first, it is necessary to recall that the human brain, with its associated mind, is a stupefying complex organ. It has been said that it is the most complex thing in the universe, and some people have doubted that we are clever enough to understand it. Reductive biologism, the concept behind biological psychiatry [1], argues that what we regard as "mind" can be fully explained with no loss of meaning by a full understanding of the physiology of the brain. That is, it attempts to explain the mind away, rather as we explained phlogiston away, by showing that the theory (of phlogiston or of mind) is a false construct, an unnecessary and misleading entity which leads us away from a proper account of the appearances. My case is that there cannot be a non-mentalist psychology, meaning biological psychiatry fails its first test [2]. We must take mental phenomena seriously [3] and one of the features to be taken seriously is malfunction of the mind, the province of psychiatry. An essential test for any theory of mind is whether it can account for the phenomena of mental disorder. There has never been a rational, testable model of mental disorder which accepted the full phenomena of mind and did not attempt to "explain them away." However, in saying we know nothing about conscious experience, I am not attempting to explain it away.

7-2. The Other Half of Mind

For several reasons, I have not given any attention to the "other mind," the realm of conscious experience. In the first place, this model is about causal efficacy, and there is no reason to believe the inner experiential realm of perception (including emotion and sensation) has any direct role in the causation of behavior. So far, there is every reason to suppose we can give an adequate explanation of behavior without needing to rely on this aspect of mental life. Secondly, and perhaps more to the point, I don't know how to start explaining conscious experience. In order to understand cognitive function, we disassemble it according to Turing's approach. However, when it comes to dismantling conscious experience into its constituent parts, we are rather like a naked man trapped inside a large, oiled fish bowl: every time he tries to climb out, he slides back to where he started. In the previous work, I suggested the possibility that the brain computes a virtual world or virtual (mental) machine by a subtle, recursive reprocessing of the basic sensory data in real time, but that this is causally ineffective in the generation of behavior [2]. This concept depends on the analogy of the programs used by architects and video games, which give a three-dimensional view of a scene. The operator can swap back and forth between internal and external views of a building, as the viewer is "walked" through and around it. By jumping back and forth between the two views, internal and external, it may be possible to invoke the illusion that there is an observer. However, this notion causes a problem for a theory that relies on the evolutionary perspective. There seems little doubt that when a chimp looks at a banana I am holding, he sees exactly the same thing as I see. There is no reason to believe that the full conscious experience of vision arose at the time *Homo sapiens* first scuttled across the veldt. That would fly in the face of everything we know of evolution [4]. But if the conscious realm is causally ineffective, how has it persisted throughout our phylogeny?

The answer may be that the conscious or experiential realm is, in fact, essential for our survival as it functions as the gateway to memory. We use our senses to attend to the world around us, but the great majority of the daily sensory input is filtered and disregarded because it is not interesting (e.g. inedible, not on heat, not dangerous, etc). We are barely aware of the great majority of this material and, shortly after, cannot recall it. However, when we attend to something, it becomes part of the conscious realm and this is the only material we can remember later. That is, attending to something brings it into the conscious experience and this is the means or gateway by which it can enter memory. This may explain why conscious experience persists when it doesn't appear to have a measurable function. In fact, it has a function, but only as part of another, essential function, memory. Granted, this is a rather inefficient system but so is human reproduction: if a system works, it will allow the species to prosper until something better comes along. Given the enormous biological investment in our sensory systems, and given their efficacy in conveying a highly accurate impression of the external world, any improvement would require such a vast mutation that it probably wouldn't be compatible with human life as we know it.

This is all I have to offer about the realm of conscious experience, but it isn't all we need to say. One day, somebody will show how to dismantle experience into its atomic elements, and then we will really have a model of mind. However, half a mind is better than no mind, so if somebody says "I'm of half a mind to whack you," he's telling the truth.

7-3. Nature vs. Nurture, Emotions vs. Rules

7-3 (a). Preparedness

Behavior is governed partly by what we have explicitly learned (education, socialization) and partly by what we have implicitly learned (personality). However, that is not all of it. For example, my daughter's birthday is at the beginning of the monsoonal season in Darwin. Every year, the beginning of the rain brings out lots of animals that have been hiding from the heat. Just after she turned two, I found a giant tree frog which is a large, brilliant leaf-green frog which, even for frogs, is of a placid disposition. As she had never seen one, I picked it up and took it to her to show her but she gave a little scream and pulled away. Her brother was happy to pick it up but she wouldn't go near it. A few weeks later, I found a young bandicoot, which is a small marsupial about the size of a puppy. Even though she had never seen one and we didn't have any pets then, she was immediately happy to see it, smiling and reaching out to pat it. Why? How is it that two animals she had never seen could cause such differing responses? The answer is that we know more than the sum total of what we have learned. We arrive equipped with a system of knowledge which is part of our biological heritage as higher primates.

The tendency for people to develop phobias about particular classes of stimuli has long been known. In the 1960s and '70s, the psychologist, Martin Seligman, developed the notion that, by virtue of our evolutionary heritage, we are biologically "prepared" to develop excessive fears of certain objects in the environment. That is, some things we come across are scarier than others. Lengthy research since then has confirmed that our fears are not equipotent, which is what classical behaviorism predicted, but we selectively discern certain potentially dangerous objects in the environment and respond to them with an exaggerated fear reaction. Furthermore, this tendency is so powerful that it can even be found in people who have never seen the objects they fear. Once exposed, they rapidly develop intense fear states which are highly resistant to extinction or retraining. The best studied example is snakes. Oehman and Mineka have shown that snake fear is universal in humans and equally as powerful in all other primates studied [8]. They concluded: "....snake stimuli are strongly and widely associated with fear in humans and other primates and ...fear of snakes is relatively independent of conscious cognition." Learning to fear snakes and responding to the animals does not require cortical processing. It appears that the distinctive features of snakes are selectively perceived in a neutral or even deliberately confusing setting. These features directly trigger the subcortical fear centers in the brain. That is, we are programmed to detect and respond to snakes without thinking. This is the "other half" of cognition, the innate cognitive system (ICS) which we share with other primates.

The principal is that we are born with a powerful tendency to avoid certain features of the environment which are likely to be dangerous. So, we fear darkness more than we fear light, we are more wary of big, scowling men than we are of whimpering children, and we are selectively repelled by certain sights and smells and attracted by others. In evolutionary terms, we can readily understand this: a tendency to avoid dangerous situations will be transmitted to the next generation just because people who don't fear snakes or dark caves are not likely to leave a next generation.

Psychologists have studied this phenomenon in considerable depth (see Oehman and Mineka for references) but have focused their attention on the fear side of the equation. My interest lies in the cognitive processes which necessarily precede the fear response: an innate fear of snakes is not much use to a blind man. What is it that allows us to recognize a snake in a field of scrub and tumbled boulders? There is a crucially important general principle at work in this specific example, one which we ignore at our peril.

7-3 (b). A cognitive basis to preparedness

I have outlined a model of cognitive function in which the sensory input undergoes a functional split. A person looking at a flower (which psychologists tend to use as a non-threatening stimulus) has two subsequent mental events. One is an experience of something colorful and attractive while the other consists of information as to what the object is and where it is, etc. The knowledge state is processed rapidly and silently to form the basis for subsequent, selective action. However, there is something about many objects or settings which automatically predisposes us to respond in certain protective ways. The knowledge state they generate is not neutral, but is programmed to incline us to particular responses even when we may not want to. That is, we are inclined to certain actions by our nature as human beings, not by our experience as individuals. These types of actions are mostly immediate, crude and unselective responses to certain classes of events or objects which, almost without fail, are geared toward ensuring survival. At one end, we have impulses such as the sex drive. Sexual orientation is unquestionably in place before first sexual experience. Similarly, the impulse to nurture small things with big foreheads and snub noses which make whimpering noises is hard to resist. A baby's squealing selectively agitates adults. We form lasting bonds, not just with other humans but also with things and places, and threats to those bonds are powerfully frightening. Our capacity to form cooperative communities has almost certainly been a major factor in our spreading to populate the globe. On an individual basis, young men in particular are highly competitive and will fight to the death rather than face humiliation of defeat. Unlike other animals, we don't just fight for food and mates but dominance itself—and freedom from domination.

Cognitively, certain essential features of a snake provoke the fear response. For example, we don't need to see its eyes to know to keep away. It is the form of a long, slender thing writhing slowly in coils that is frightening, and it is exactly these features which are easy to recognize just because they stimulate the retinal receptors maximally. Everybody is familiar with the strobe lights on police cars. These are effective just because they stimulate the peripheral retinal on-off receptors at their maximal rate. Anything slower or faster than about 12Hz is less effective in attracting attention. There is no cognitive intermediation; the retinal receptors are directly connected to the brainstem centers subserving the orienting reflex. As soon as the receptors are stimulated, we turn toward the light, just as monkeys do, and it takes a powerful determination not to respond. The same principle of "mindless apprehension" applies to the snake. Sinusoidal movements are highly effective in activating retinal edge detectors (which are just aligned on-off detectors), which provokes a particular pattern of input in the optic nerves. At some early stage in the processing of this input, certainly well before it reaches the cortex, this pattern causes signals to be sent directly to the limbic structures subserving the arousal response. Even before the person is fully aware of what is happening, he is responding with a sudden burst of fear and immediate withdrawal. Pattern recognition software in a desktop computer can easily reproduce effect. There is no need to invoke a mind in this type of response.

The "crucially important general principle" in this example is the notion of unwilled subcortical data processing which directly provokes behavioral responses by means of emotional activation. Taken together, this amounts to an innate cognitive system, in contrast with the adaptive cognitive system. Granted, a fear of snakes is a bit extreme in that it is an "all-or-none" response but it serves to illustrate the general point of what used to be called "instinctive responses." By this, I mean an unreasoned, goal-directed, emotion-based behavioral response to an external event which occurs before there can be effective reflection. It isn't all bad: is the sense of humor is a very good example. A person laughs before he has time to consider whether he should. Sexual arousal is innate in the sense that it is not learned, either explicitly or implicitly. Most of what we would consider bad or destructive human behavior has its origins in this vast, primitive system but so does a lot of behavior which is essential to survival.

7-3 (c). Objections to evolutionary cognitivism

A potential objection is that this is just a clever way of pulling what was formerly known as "reflex behavior" into the cognitive net, of evading the claims of reductive biologism by relabeling their discoveries as mentalist. I don't believe this is a valid objection. It should be quite clear that I am not denying the role of monosynaptic reflexes such as the knee jerk or the corneal reflex. Similarly, I have no problem with the fundamentally biological nature of, say, the immune response or the physiological control of blood pressure. With monosynaptic reflex arcs, the data input does not reach the brain proper but stays in the peripheries, and is not modified or transformed in any appreciable way. It is a simple matter of a one-to-one relationship between sensory input and behavioral output, with little or no modification of the signal. Unlike the responses mediated by the innate cognitive system, tendon reflexes are not an inclination to respond. A person can learn to love snakes but he cannot stop his knee jerk. In the ICS, a complex informational input is processed and then becomes the basis for a graded, directed, emotionally-driven behavioral routine which varies according to the immediate circumstances. However, when compared with the full subtlety of the adaptive cognitive system, behavioral responses mediated by the ICS are crude and often maladaptive.

Similarly, there is no parallel between cognition and the chemically-mediated cellular responses of even the most complex physiological systems. For a start, hormonal and cell-based control systems do not involve neuronal transmission of sensory input. There is no date-processing, so they cannot be considered to be part of the cognitive system in any way. The body's many control systems, including such complex cases as the portal systems of the pituitary [9, p195-6], have a perfectly rational explanation in physicochemical terms. The causative loops in these two examples are physically complete in themselves and their explanation does not rely on any notion of mentality or meaning. That is, they are constrained by the laws of thermodynamics, not the rules of semantics. Because of this, I do not accept the objection as having any conviction.

7-3 (d). The innate cognitive system as human nature

As mentioned, the mechanism of the ICS is relatively simple: with minimal processing, the current sensory input to the brain is directed to the emotional systems and thence to behavioral effector systems. By this means, the sensory input exerts powerful effects over emotional activity, in turn dramatically increasing the probability of certain behaviors. Taken together, these behaviors are roughly what we know as human nature. There is a vast body of observational and experimental evidence to support this concept. Anybody who wants to know about human nature should start with our nearer relatives, the great apes and communal primates such as baboons. What we see about them is more or less what our old friend, the visiting anthropologist from Mars, would see about us. Thus, the Martian visitor would report that we are social creatures whose need for social bonding is so strong that children deprived of it will usually die. Within our social groups, we quickly form unstable dominance hierarchies. These are violently obvious in young adult males, and subtly obvious in all other members of *H. sapiens.* Just like baboons, we are xenophobic and have strong territorial and acquisitive drives. We show play behavior and aggression, we are comforted by the familiar yet we are incurably curious; we like to explore but we resist change. In short, we are riven by a mass of contradictions.

These are the behavioral features usually known as "human nature," but they are in fact higher primate nature because most of our hairier relatives show them too. Unfortunately, a lot of our worst behavior seems to result from this system but we wouldn't be here if we didn't have something like it. The survival value of the innate cognitive system is beyond doubt but it certainly does not run by "sweet reason." Even lofty emotions such as the sense of justice may have their roots in the ICS. A sense of satisfaction over somebody getting his "just desserts" may be no more rational than the pleasure of seeing a competitor (for territory, sexual partners, or dominance) toppled by "the rules."

The adaptive cognitive system allows precise, finely attuned responses to subtle features in the environment. The individual is able to look at the world and decide exactly how he wishes to go about exploiting it to his advantage. In particular, it permits the notion of rules as binding injunctions on group behavior, subjecting the innate, visceral cognitive functions to a higher control, thereby allowing the development of stable societies. The difference between the adaptive and innate cognitive systems is that the, while the ICS is more or less directly connected to emotional centers, the ACS works through logic gates interposed between sensory input and behavioral output. It allows us to see relationships, to count and, above all, to develop a sense of other people as creatures with similar minds whose intentions can be guessed with sufficient accuracy to save one's life. This is our rational side, but most of the trouble we cause ourselves is because the innate cognitive system is not well-controlled. Worse, we are able to convince ourselves we are acting from noble motives even when our actions are actually under the control of the emotion-driven innate cognitive system.

The question of how mental life starts is very important. Newborn babies don't have much cognitive capacity at all but, within a few weeks or months, they can selectively respond to familiar faces and voices, to smiles and scowls, and let the world know about it. This is invariable: a child who doesn't show it is in serious trouble. A child's intellectual capacity develops through a series of well-recognized stages until, by about 18-24 months, he is starting to show individualized responses to the world. The biocognitive model proposes that, by this stage, the brain is developing the specific neuronal connections I have termed logic gates. Whereas previously, the child was driven by his genetic endowment as a primate, the two year old is now able to learn and begin to take control of his destiny. Gradually, the child's wants, fears (and furies) begin to over-ride his innate dispositions. The adaptive cognitive system (ACS) develops out of and eventually dominates the ICS, but the primitive innate system is never very far away.

Rules are critical to our survival as a species. Before we can know anything, we have to have rules but, before we can have rules, we must have a brain that can deal with logical abstractions. Without our capacity to elaborate rule-governed behavior, including speech, we would not be able to develop cooperative behavior, such as group hunting. Before we can be *Homo sapiens,* the knowing creature, we have to be *Homo nomotheticus,* the Rule-Giver. However, there must be no doubt that, as social animals with an adaptive cognitive system, we develop the rules we want. Social rules are not innate but are acquired, and not always for the reasons given. In the Darwinian sense, every rule in society benefits somebody. In ordinary life, we often do not distinguish between the effects of the innate and the adaptive cognitive systems, but take them as one and the same thing. This is wrong:

they are ontologically and anatomically different, and we cannot ignore those differences. The Cold War arms race was a good example of how the adaptive cognitive system can be subverted to work for the innate system. Men used their intellects to devise weapons of aggression of vast power and complexity without ever asking the larger question of what they thought they were doing. Rules are the basis of language, of civil society and, of course, of science but we need to distinguish very clearly between the formal rules of the adaptive cognitive system and the crude, rule-like reactions of the ICS.

Without a rapidly adapting cognitive system which allows us to profit from experience and to devise and change our plans on the run, we would have followed *H. erectus* into oblivion. However, unless we use the adaptive system to bring the innate cognitive system under better control, we may yet go the little chap's way.

7-3 (e). Traditional notions of human nature and the biocognitive model

Fascinating though the task would be, it is not feasible to attempt a detailed account of the many versions of human nature throughout the ages. Instead, I will compare my model with two major systems of belief, Christianity and Marxism, and the recent version advocated by the behaviorists. Since I have already alluded to the role of religious beliefs in generating support for biological psychiatry, it is appropriate to specify the biocognitive account of human nature in order to prevent misunderstanding.

The classic Christian concept of human nature is part of a closed ontological system, meaning it offers accounts of the nature of the universe, of humanity's place in the universe, of the nature of mankind's problems and a remedy for those problems. That is, it is formally classified as an ideology. Stevenson [10] argues further that all ideologies are typified by two epistemological features. First, its believers can always find something in the belief system that allows them to negate criticism. In Popper's terms, they can immunize their theory against refutation. Secondly, the believer can always find some means in the theory or belief system that allows him, not just to deny the critic's complaints, but to attack him, verbally, if not physically. A third point he doesn't emphasize is that, if anybody strays from the path, it is not the fault of the belief system but of the individual himself. There is nothing the individual can do which will refute the belief system as it is not just without fault but is incapable of being wrong. The belief system comes from an authority which cannot be questioned so, if anybody does so, he is necessarily wrong by virtue of his own willfulness, and sanctions apply.

For Western Christians, the universe is the creation of an omnipotent, omniscient God. While early Christians saw the whole thing as a mystery, by the Enlightenment, the educated view (and the one with which we are familiar) was that the universe was a marvelous machine, silently ticking over according to precisely defined mathematical rules which were part of Creation. The astounding way the universe fitted together was taken as evidence of divine design. Having set His machine in motion, God was able to take a less involved role and probably didn't interfere from moment to moment as the Old Testament seemed to indicate. Man (and, as a second thought, woman) was the result of a special and deliberate act of creation intended to yield a being halfway between angels and animals, i.e. physically of the world but with an immortal soul which was not part of the material universe. The purpose of humans was to love God and please him by doing his will; by acts of willful folly, man (encouraged by woman) strayed from God's intended path and was forced to leave the wonderful setting God had made for this vale of tears. By acknowledging his wrongdoing and begging forgiveness, humans could once again be at one with their Creator and live in eternal bliss. Thus, we have the nature of the universe, humanity's place in it, a diagnosis of what went wrong and a prescription to rectify those wrongs.

For the intellectually curious, this is quite a good ontology as it allows people to explore not just the world itself (to acquaint people with the vast wonder of God's creation) but to probe its inner workings, and not just of the world but of humans themselves. This can be done because there is no risk of treading on forbidden ground, as it were. The soul is God's territory alone but, because it is immaterial, there is nothing we can do to probe its mysteries as our tools are wholly of the material realm. So we can potter around in the blood and mud because its fate is that, one day, it will turn to dust; anyway, it isn't divine in nature so who really cares? So scientists and explorers could be good materialists all week, yet still go to church on Sundays and feel no contradiction in doing so.

Despite the battering it has taken over the past twenty years, the Marxist view is still very influential, and not just among people who claim to be Marxists. This is an avowedly atheistic, materialist stance. Marx was adamantly opposed to religion, which he saw as a blinding distraction from human reality. The nature of the universe is material, with no room for magical tricks like immortal souls. Therefore, he did not see humans as having a purpose, as Christians do: people simply are, and that is that. Humans wish to be happy and self-fulfilled but are alienated from their creative and productive selves by the need to earn a living in a particular social system. Societies are driven by the need for humans to achieve happiness and therefore must progress toward the goal of the maximum satisfaction for the greatest number of people. The ultimate goal he saw was that society would eventually and inevitably reach a state in which all people felt able to express themselves in the absence of fear—fear of want, fear of suppression and of the future, etc. His diagnosis was the alienation and his remedy the rapid progress of society toward the utopian future. Again, criticism could be neutered by the view that only a person who opposes human advancement could object to the Marxist view, meaning those who were gaining most from the oppressive state of the society and stood to lose most by an equitable social system. Hence the violent antipathy of the Marxists for their enemies but, in this respect, they were really no different from Christians throughout most of their history.

The biocognitive model is not in the same league as these examples. First, it is cast in the materialist ontology, but it merely borrows this and has not contributed to it in any significant fashion. Granted, this model expands the realm of materialism to include not just matter and energy but the informational states that control them but this is not new. It does not contradict any of the principles that govern matter and energy. Secondly, it offers a view of human nature but this is strictly empirical and can be changed according to the evidence. In this respect, it differs very dramatically from the two models given above, which cannot be questioned without throwing doubt on the whole edifice. Marxism is incompatible with the notion that humans have eternal souls while Christianity cannot coexist with a doctrine that denies the existence of a Creator. The biocognitive model simply says that, for the purposes of discussion, immaterial souls do not exist. There may in fact be a divinity but the materialist theory is sufficient in itself to account for all known observations and divinities are superfluous. Since it gives a complete explanatory account of all behavior, there is no need for a soul even though souls may actually exist.

It is on the next point, the diagnosis of what is wrong with humans, that the biocognitive model definitely parts company with Christianity and Marxism. There is nothing wrong with humans. This model is strictly empirical, and empiricism makes no moral claims. Morality and empiricism exist in different realms of discourse. As George Orwell noted in another context, they are like a sausage and a rose: their purposes do not intersect. Claims that there is something wrong with human life depend on the claimant having access to privileged information regarding its goals and direction, whereas the materialist ontology exists without goals. So, humans can be as good or as bad, as happy or as unhappy as they like but that does not imply any ontological fracture lines. There are no goals in a materialist playing field. Mental disorder is a reality but it has no probitive value, it is not a question of right or wrong any more than a broken leg has a moral value (outside Erewhon, of course). Humans can bumble ahead, assembling either a lasting, sustainable and equitable civilization or they can engineer their own extinction but that is for them to decide as their existence serves no larger purpose, nor are they driven in a direction ordained by the biocognitive model. This model is therefore not an ideology and no moral injunctions can be derived from it.

Just for interest, it is worth applying the above tests to the reductionist model of biological psychiatry. Its larger ontology is materialist but, as I have shown, there is an inherent contradiction as theirs is a very restricted model of materialism. It does not give an account of essential psychological values such as religion. It claims that psychological values can be reduced to material objects but that is rather silly as electrons have no minds in which values can inhere. Biological reductionism does not give an account of human nature. However, I would say that this is mainly due to lack of intellectual curiosity among biological psychiatrists than because they have no material. If they wished, they could simply say that human nature is just a turbo-charged version of higher primate nature and they would be on safe ground, but they have been so obsessed with finding biochemical abnormalities that they have neglected seeing that their model must fit with other fields of empirical science. This leads to their universal diagnosis, that everything wrong with humans is a biochemical imbalance of the brain, and to their universal prescription, drugs. I would say that this entails a contradiction, as it implies they know what behavior would allow them to say when a person's brain is chemically balanced, and that is nonsensical. It is nonsensical because human behavior is dimensionally distributed, not categorically, whereas chemical imbalances of the brain are a category of disorder, not a dimension. In particular, biological psychiatry does not have a theoretical basis that would allow a distinction to be drawn between "normal but unpleasant or stupid behavior" and "pathological behavior." A lot of what is called deviant behavior is just an extreme variant of normal behavior, or even normal behavior in abnormal situations. For example, mowing people down with a machine gun is normal in war but undesirable in civilian life. In fact, much of the behavior biological psychiatry deems "mental illness" is a result of the innate cognitive system (human nature) working perfectly normally. It is for this reason that I believe biological psychiatry lurches perilously close to being an ideology (values masquerading as objectivity), not an empirical science, and that is dangerous (which is itself an irreducible value judgment).

7-4. A Fragile Logic Machine: Confusion and Dementia

There now doesn't seem much doubt that the brain functions as a high-speed data processor, using (at least in part) well-known principles which, especially over the last fifty or so years, have been exploited very successfully in all fields of science. As neurophysiology probes deeper into the brain's molecular function, its true complexity is becoming increasingly apparent to us. Despite its complexity, our daily experience of going about life tends to suggest the brain is pretty tough. Without any particular attention from us, it does its job day in, day out, and we don't have to worry about it. However, psychiatrists have always known is that it malfunctions rather more easily than many people would like to admit. We know that when the lights go out in a medical ward, apparently rational people start to talk to long-dead relatives, or get out of bed saying they have to put the cat out. Confusional states are extremely common. With as little as sixty hours of sleep deprivation, healthy people begin to hallucinate but, for very sick people, it is much less, perhaps only a few hours. Drugs, both legal and illegal, readily and predictably induce disturbances of contact with reality, as do fevers, general metabolic disturbances, concussion etc. These effects are amplified if there is a mild degree of diffuse brain damage that would not normally be evident except on specialized testing. This is because the brain is not "pretty tough," it only seems that way. It operates within very narrow physiological limits of temperature, oxygen and glucose supply, etc., and the moment those limits are breached, the brain's minutely controlled function begins to deviate from normal. This is manifest as confusion and disorientation.

Since the mind is the most complex brain function, which depends not only on the integrity of the brain itself but also upon its own internal consistency, then any deviation in brain function will be magnified in its effect on mental function. Initially, this is seen as a mild confusion, starting perhaps as just a few slips in words or social mistakes, then spreading to involve judgment, social awareness, memory, planning and eventually language, etc. At its extreme, the confused person is hallucinated and often develops transient delusional beliefs, some as obvious attempts to rationalize the experiences ("I know you're hiding my brother in that room, I heard him calling me last night"), some as latent personality factors ("You've been having an affair, I saw you talking to that woman"), while some arise *de novo*.

This model dictates that the correct approach to confusional states is to look at the brain as a highly complex organ, acquitting a myriad functions in a distributed, modular pattern by integrated, high-speed processing of data derived from a broad range of internal and external sources. Fevers, drugs, concussion, marginal oxygenation or a falling BSL etc. will cause widespread, minor malfunctions of the neuronal logic gates on which the whole enterprise depends. At first, these will have subtle effects, barely noticeable to anybody who doesn't know the patient well, but they will intensify rapidly as his condition deteriorates. It is most important to remember that the confusional process can become self-reinforcing. Fear and anger (perhaps caused by the hallucinatory or delusional experiences) can cause excessive arousal which further interferes with the failing brain's function. The clinical picture of confusion is characteristic but it can be understood through a proper appreciation of brain function. This principle also applies to early dementia and to focal brain damage [5]. As an analogy, an ordinary desk-top computer will start to malfunction if it gets too hot, or it if is operated in a dusty or humid atmosphere. If it already has a minor hardware problem, then this problem will be magnified by the effects of high temperature, etc.

Thus, as the damage accumulates, there will be a gradual loss of function, starting with the most complex and demanding, meaning highest order computations. These will involve the capacity to extract subtle cues from the environment, apprehending their furthest reaching significance, and then to integrate them with a range of demands from a variety of sources. Because there will be isolated failures of individual neurons in the complex networks which subserve these functions, the effects of brain illness will first become visible as small impairments of judgment. Gradually, as the confusional state affects more and more of the brain, these defects will spread until the person is making coarse assessments and interpreting them in line with the most basic, defensive stances, essentially fearful withdrawal or the paranoid view. Dementia, in which there is a loss of brain substance and the associated mental functions, will lead to the person relying on increasingly basic rules of life as more and more functions deteriorate. Eventually, the affected individual will have only his most basic functional rules left, leaving a caricature of his former personality and intellectual abilities. He will lose the ability to look ahead and see the consequences of his actions, meaning his behavior will be crude and unmodified, with primitive, unconsidered responses to situations he once would have managed with subtlety and tact.

While we now have some idea of the mechanism by which the mind is generated, we don't know, and may never know, the exact nature of the codes that subserve our cognitive processes. We do know that mental function takes place at a level beneath that of the spoken languages, that, for example, decisions are made at a non-verbal level (probably in the prefrontal cortex) and are then translated into speech by other centers [5, 6]. There are in fact two levels of codes, the codes the brain uses to generate the mind, and the codes by which the mind operates which allow it to control the brain. The brain's codes are far beyond us: as yet, we have no technology that would allow us to look at a functioning neuron and say: "Oh yes, that's signaling it would like white tea with no sugar." The mind's codes, however, are probably forever beyond us as a matter of principle, not technology. Whether we will ever know any of these codes is moot but I doubt psychiatrists need to know. We don't have to know what goes on between a person hearing a word and his behavioral response, all we need to know is that there is a consistent, rational relationship. We can be sure that the codes are simple and robust and, as long as the brain is physically healthy, they do their job remarkably well.

7-5. Personality in The Cognitive Model

The cognitive model of mind generates the notion that personality just is the set of core beliefs and rules by which a person runs his life [2]. To summarize: personality is the sum total of the interactions between an individual and his environment. However, this is a clumsy definition, so we shorten it to read: personality is the total of the habitual interactions between an individual and his environment in the stable, adult mode of behavior. Because we are interested in the differences between individuals, the definition excludes socially-determined behaviors including language (just because you and I both speak English doesn't mean we have the same personality), convention and customs, etc. That is, we exclude explicitly-learned material. The other major exclusion is intellect. Personality is independent of intellect: we are not talking about whether a person can solve sums, only whether he approaches them methodically or flies into a rage. We want to find the set of behavioral rules which determine how each individual tackles his day, independent of what he has been taught, where he is and so on. We are looking for the underlying rules which continue to operate more or less regardless of his circumstances but which color his behavior so he can be distinguished from his neighbors.

This is still a boring definition. Describing behavior does not explain it, and our interest in personality lies in having some account of the hidden mechanisms that generate observable behavior. The value of the term personality is heuristic: we want to use it to make worthwhile predictions about a person, and the best way known of saying something reliable about a person's future conduct is to look at his past conduct. An individual's "habitual interactions in the stable adult mode of behavior" don't change very much at all. An aggressive teenager is likely to be an aggressive adult; a shy and insecure young man will never be a great social success in his forties; a tidy and methodical recruit to the army will most likely be a rigid and ritualistic soldier by the time he marches off to the old soldiers' home. We readily identify behavioral regularities, and something regular is producing these regularities, some unseen mechanism is generating them, and that unseen regulating principle is what we call personality. In order to understand it better and, if possible, to rectify its shortcomings, we need to know the nature of the "unseen regulating principle called personality."

In the cognitive model, behavior is generated by the computation of data inputs according to pre-existing instructions coded into memory, or rules. It has to be this way otherwise behavior would be chaotic and unpredictable. The interesting rules are the ones we can't access easily:

> Q: "Why did you laugh when that man fell over?"
> A: "I don't know, it just struck me as funny."
> Q: "Why did you leave your job?"
> A: "I felt the other people were angry at me for asking questions."
> Q: "Why did you yell at your children?"

A: "I just got so sick of the mess they make."
Q: "Why did you threaten your girlfriend?"
A: "I thought she was seeing somebody behind my back."
Q: "Why do you take drugs?"
A: "I just can't cope without them."

We can now define personality as the sum total of implicit, behaviorally-effective rules which serve to distinguish the individual's observable behavior from his neighbors'. Some people might object to the idea that the rules must be implicit as the obsessional personality will demand that everything be in its place, but he can't explain why he believes this. Ask him: "Why does everything have to be so tidy?" and you will get only a blank stare. Push him, and he will eventually be reduced to saying: "That's how I want it because I get upset if it isn't tidy."

Personality is the sum total of the cognitive rules which govern a person's life. If those rules are consistent and mesh neatly with the rules of society, then we would say the person has a normal personality. Rules can, however, be internally inconsistent, causing erratic behavior or leading the person to perform well below the level his physical and intellectual resources would suggest. Similarly, if the rules provoke excessive emotional responses to everyday events or bring the person into conflict with society, then we would say he has a personality disorder. Again, this model states unequivocally that there is no suggestion of a physical brain disorder as the basis of personality disorder. It is the subject's belief system that is faulty, not the cerebral machinery that implements his belief system. That is to say, when people respond with excessive anxiety to otherwise neutral events in the environment, their brains are working perfectly well. There is no "chemical imbalance of the brain," just a maladaptive rule of life buried somewhere in the subject's cognitive apparatus. This is why someone can show appalling behavior in one part of life but be charming and rule-abiding in another: that just is his set of rules.

It follows that the numbers of rules that can influence a person's can behavior is practically unlimited. Year after year, daily experience generates a huge range of generalizations from the very broadest to the most specific and trivial. There is no limit and certainly no guarantee that, if two people are exposed to the same situation, they will both derive the same conclusions from it. Conversely, the same behavioral patterns in two people can have entirely different motivations. One person is fanatically tidy for fear of getting into trouble while his neighbor may show exactly the same pattern as a means of dominating people. At any time, there may be many different rules contributing to a particular behavioral outcome. As Freud said, all behavior is over-determined, as there can be only one action regardless of the numbers of rules that have had a role in shaping it. It is important not to make the mistake of believing that there is a single motivating factor behind each class of behaviors. For example, the cluster of behaviors seen in aggressive personalities can be based in a need to dominate, a fear of being dominated or humiliated, a sense of being insignificant, a sense of persecution, an excessive startle response and so on. Avoidant behavior can be based in a sense of superiority, a fear of being seen inferior through making mistakes or not knowing how to act, a disinterest in other people, an excessive interest in matters of the intellect, a fear of the natural or the social world, etc.

When assessing personality, the usual approach is to ask a wide range of questions and extract their common features. Psychometric assessment of the personality simply applies statistical techniques to this process to standardize the questions and cluster the answers so that there is rough agreement that the tests are assessing much the same behaviors against similar standards. However, most tests do not look beyond the surface. Some, like the MMPI, have been used so widely and for so long that they can yield a great deal of information about unsuspected correlations among the classes of behaviors but they are still not based in a model of mind. The describe behavior, clustering it into useful groups, but they do not explain the subject's implicit rules, the hidden generative mechanisms of that behavior.

7-6. Conclusion

It would be convenient to refer to Chalmers' model of the duality of mind as, say, the "bicameral theory of mind," but this would encourage people to think in terms of boxes. Boxes have things "in" them and observers to look "at" them, which is entirely the wrong approach as it leads to the infinite regress of the Cartesian model. I prefer to talk of the biocognitive model as a "biphasic model of mind," meaning dual aspects of a virtual entity. It is virtual, because mental functions are not of and never can be reduced to the physical realm, and its two aspects, the experiential realm and the knowledge state, are fundamentally different ways of utilizing the same data input. These functions coexist in time and quite possibly in the space of the same neural networks, but they are causally separate and do not interfere with each other, and probably don't even interact. Each amounts to a fully-functional virtual machine in its own right derived, presumably, from different forms of data processing. Perhaps we should start to think of the mind in terms of a cluster of virtual entities running in relative functional isolation.

While the workings of the experiential realm remain beyond our grasp, the knowledge state seems amenable to explanation in familiar terms. For psychiatry, this is of cardinal importance as the informational realm determines behavior, including the emotional state. Empirically, the knowledge realm is composed of two closely-related cognitive systems. The older system is the innate cognitive system which we share, to a greater or lesser extent, with other higher primates. This is the emotive or visceral side of life, the fun bit as well as the dangerous bit. This system is common to all humans and forms the greater part of what we call human nature. Because it is primarily genetically determined, its influence almost certainly varies according to a normal distribution, and it would therefore account for part of the usual variation in temperament or character between individuals. The more recent part, the adaptive cognitive system, further divides into two functionally distinct parts, the implicit and the explicit systems. These two systems are intimately related and account for the rest of the variation in temperament, especially the implicit system.

This model offers an explanation of the nature of the cerebral systems which give rise to observable behavior, including speech and emotion. If correct, it would form the basis of an integrated system of knowledge, as outlined in the diagram. While it leads to a theory of morality, it has no moral content of its own, which safeguards against any attempt to turn it into an ideology. It says that humans are as they are, that there is no perfect state or utopian idea toward which they are progressing. It says, for example, that we are compelled to form emotional bonds by our genetic heritage just because this feels better than isolation, and that this is normal. The converse is that breaking those bonds is necessarily going to lead to unhappiness, and that this is also normal. As long as there are human bonds, there will be humans grieving the loss of those bonds, and there is no utopia in which this will ever be different. Grief is unavoidable, just because it is programmed into us, part of the human condition, and no diets or massages, chants or revolutions will ever alter our DNA. Distress is immanent. Only a charlatan would claim otherwise, and only a fool would believe him.

Common Observation	Evolutionary Theory	Philosophy of mind and of science	Cognitive neuroscience	Ethology, anthropology, sociology

PROPOSED SOLUTION TO THE MIND-BODY PROBLEM

Prohibits the supernatural **and** fanatical religion.

Restricts pharmacy **Denies** fringe medicine

THEORY OF MIND
(Perception, cognition, action)

Theory of Human Nature	Theory of Language	Theory of Personality	Theory of Mental Disorder

Naturalistic Theory of Morality

Theory of Epistemology

?Free Will

Theory of Personality Disorder

Theory of society

Science and technology

?Creativit

Ethical Theory of Psychiatry

Theory of Law

Art, Music

Rational Treatment

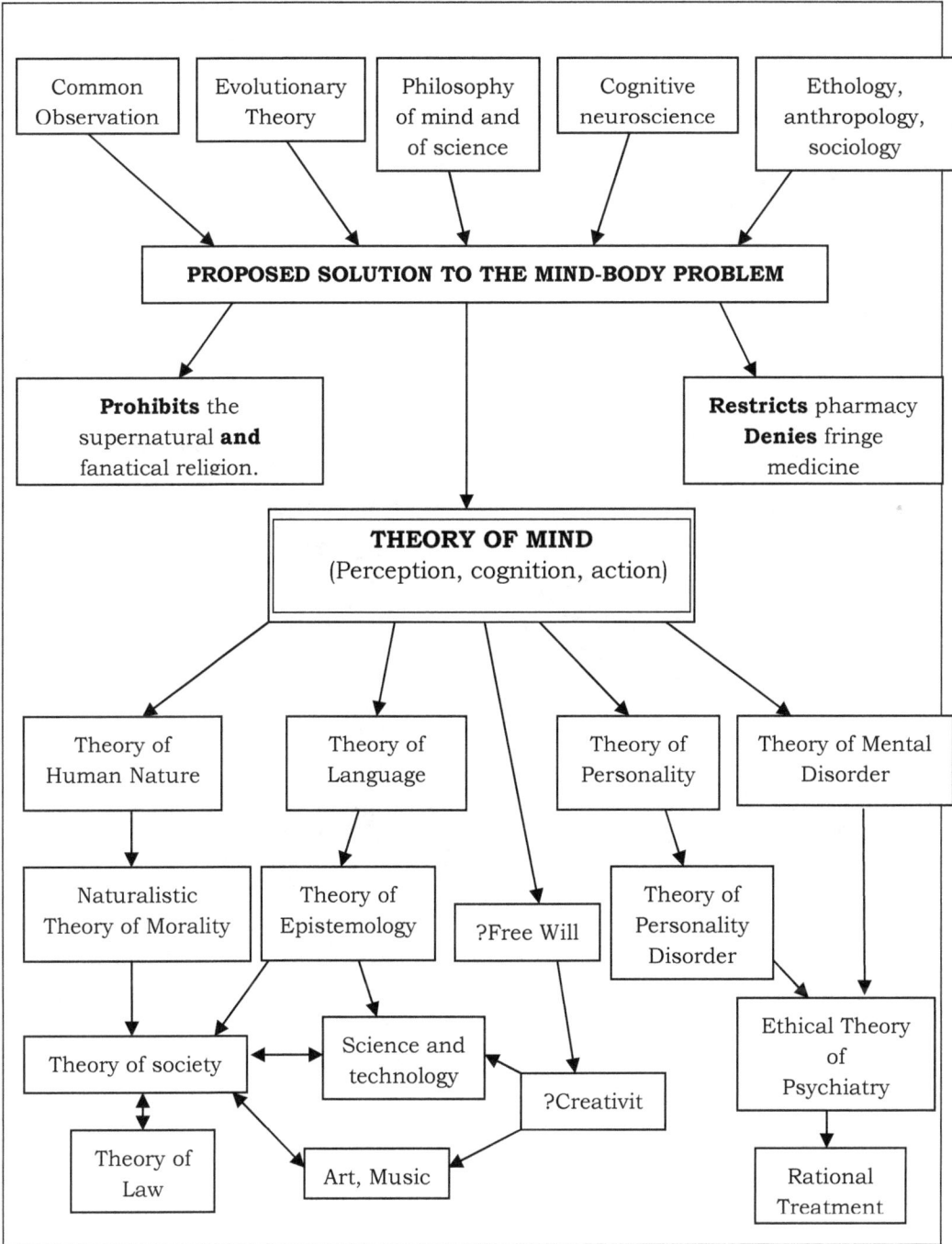

Fig. 7-1: Logical Structure of the Biocognitive Model

8 Language as a Test of the Biocognitive Model

"A myth is not a fairy story. It is the presentation of facts belonging to one category in the idioms of another. To explode a myth is not to deny the facts but to reallocate them."

Gilbert Ryle

8-1. Introduction

The 'biocognitive' model of mental disorder being developed in this and the preceding work [1] is unique in the history of psychiatry in that it offers an explanatory account of the essential features of mental disorder in the context of a larger, integrative theory of mind. Very briefly, the model begins with the common phenomena of mental life and splits them in two realms, according to the concept of natural dualism developed by the philosopher David Chalmers. These are the conscious or experiential realm, which includes sensation, emotion, etc., and the knowledge-based or decision-making realm, which Chalmers calls the psychological realm. For psychiatry, the latter half of mind is causally-significant. It functions outside conscious awareness, at high speed, generating the decisions which lead to observable behavior. The functional parallel with the concept of "mindless decision-making," pioneered by the mathematician, Alan Turing, is not just coincidental. After it has been rendered in physical form, Turing's concept leads to a non-question-begging, finite explanation of the effective mind without invoking any principles not already in use elsewhere in science.

The crucial mechanism is the concept of logic gates, without which logical processes cannot be actualized. Modern understanding of neuronal function indicates very strongly that neurons function as high-speed, multichannel logic gates. In turn, the microarchitecture of the cerebral cortex is of a form consistent with the processing and integration of very large cascades of data from a variety of sources. That the brain supports massively parallel data processing is now beyond question. Thus, if we equate the high speed, inaccessible knowledge functions of mind with the manipulation of brain-based information, we arrive at a theoretical basis of causally-effective mind-body interaction. Just as the logic gates in a child's toy control their own function, so too the neuronal logic gates control their own function, meaning body and mind are linked at this precise point. From this feature, it is possible to derive an account of mental disorder as a primary disturbance of psychological function within the context of a normal brain, i.e. there is no "chemical imbalance of the brain" in most, perhaps all, mental disorder.

However, models have to be tested against reality, and the harshest test for any model of mind is language. Language is probably the most complex human function of all. While there has been considerable progress in analyzing language as semantics, and in neurophysiology, we are not yet in a position to show how these aspects of communication are functionally related. Can the biocognitive model give an account of language which satisfies the twin notions of language as disembodied communication, and language as a brain-based function? In this chapter, I will outline a biological mechanism of language production which satisfies a number of major philosophical tests a plausible theory of language must pass.

8-2. Language Divorced from the Brain

We have a problem when we speak about language. It is utterly basic to our existence and yet we usually take it for granted. A theory of language attempts to give a rational account of what we do when we speak. A philosophy of language is a critical comparison of two or more theories of language [2]. There have been dozens of attempts at theories of language, most of them somewhat successful on one or other point, but none of them able to explain the totality of what small children can do when they are playing together.

To a large extent, each theory depends on what its author sees as the central language function. For some people, the function of language is to refer to real things in the natural world but, ten thousand times a day, we refer to things which don't seem to belong to reality as we would like to think of it. Some words refer to abstract concepts, such as goodness or loneliness, which are part of life as we understand it. Others refer to apparent entities, such as pixies and bunyips, which have no objective reality, while many concepts of science and mathematics, not to overlook economics, seem to be real enough but they are not entities in any convincing sense of the word. Other authors take questions of truth and falsity to be central to their concept of language but a very large part of human speech seems to have little to do with truth. Is it true that Darth Vader was Luke Skywalker's father? A very large part of daily language is simply fiction, while questions, greetings and other formal speech acts, emotive expressions and statements about the future don't seem to have any points of contact with the notion of truth. This seems to leave us with a theory of language that has no firm contact with reality and only a passing acquaintance with truth.

Some theorists have attempted to get around these problems by suggesting that language actually refers to ideas in the speaker's head but this immediately runs into difficulties, such as how to define ideas, or ideas with no imagery, and concepts such as negative numbers whose attached ideas prove remarkably slippery. In fact, this applies to all mentalist concepts. Under

Skinner's influence, radical behaviorists tried to avoid any references to the mental realm by insisting that language had nothing to do with mind as we normally use the term. They saw it as simply a mindless, biologically-determined process by which the environment of the verbal community shapes and maintains our responses to each other's verbal stimuli. Chomsky skewered this notion very early in its life but it refused to lie down, and several generations of psychologists believed, quite wrongly, that they "understood" the concept of *lingua sine mens*, a mindless language. It is now difficult to understand why this was the case. In brief, radical behaviorism says that children acquire language under the influence of the existing verbal community. By a process which does not involve mental intervening variables, the infant's various gurglings are gradually converted into the language of its parents. The child makes a variety of sounds (emits operants, in Skinner's terms, operants being random behaviors which operate upon the environment) to which the parents respond favorably. By selectively responding to the child's noises, the parents shape its verbal behavior more and more closely to the words they want their baby to use. By this means, the child acquires the capacity to use the mature language, all without mentalism.

There are many problems with this notion, not the least of which is that it is not true. In the first place, parental reinforcement is anything but selective. For example, the child cries. This can be for any number of reasons because infants can't do much else to register displeasure. The parents pick their baby up and soothe it. The child then stops crying and starts to look around again. According to Skinner's theory, this should not happen. Cuddling a crying child should act as a positive reinforcer for crying: by his principles, we should all be crying all the time, just because we have been strongly reinforced to do so. However, comforting the child stops it crying, which is the exact opposite of what his theory predicts: the more reinforcement it gets, the more it should cry. Secondly, parents are simply hopeless at reinforcing behavior. They are so happy to hear the infant's squawks and splutters that they reinforce baby talk very strongly. Nonetheless, and despite hearing all the wrong cues, the toddler soon begins to use complete sentences of the standard language, very often abandoning baby talk long before the doting parents do.

It is the case that babies acquire language much faster and far more selectively than Skinner's theory of operant conditioning can account for. Only a theory which credits mental intervening variables can account for this. Human infants have an innate capacity to soak up the complexity of language which chimp infants simply do not have. Radical behaviorism could not account for this. At the same time, it could not account for the way parents respond to their babies. Parents have a strong urge to pick up their children when they cry; this is powerful and universal, meaning it is innate, not acquired. Chimp parents also have the bad habit of positively reinforcing their babies' dysfunctional behavior but, despite their parents' failings, the infants soon become good chimp citizens and go on to show the same bad habits themselves. Perhaps because of these very obvious failings of the Skinnerian model, other philosophers of language have taken the view that language is just a complex social game, in which people infer the speaker's intent and signal their comprehension by giving an appropriate response. This does not appear to give creativity its due, but also begs the question of meaning. More recent attempts at a theory of language have been overtly mentalist in nature but they revive the original problem, namely, the lack of a convincing theory of mind in which to embed the function of language [3].

Neurologists have convincingly demonstrated the role of brain systems in the generation of the physical act of speech but their approach does not and cannot address the semantic content of language. The neurological act of speaking is distinct from the intentional content of language, just as the neurology of rapid movements of the hand says nothing about the contents of a note the owner of the hand has just written. This points to a critically important question for psychiatry: can the semantic content of language be reduced to a brain function? Different theories in psychiatry have responded to this question in different ways, mostly by ignoring it. For example, psycho-analysis, perhaps more than most theories, depends upon the patient's utterances to give a reliable account of intrapsychic activity. Following Freud's example, psychoanalysts, even medical analysts, took no account whatsoever of brain function. Less extreme approaches, such as Engel's biopsychosocial model [9], assume the reality of mind-brain interaction but have no means of integrating the two levels of function. Biological psychiatry, on the other hand, assumes that any and all mental functions can be reduced directly to brain functions, such that a detailed knowledge of brain function will tell all we need to know about the patient's mental life. Disturbances of mental function, such as the thought disorder of schizophrenia, are assumed to be due to a "chemical imbalance of the brain," the precise nature of which will be revealed by molecular physiology. This approach is incorrect: in principle, mental functions cannot be reduced to brain functions just because there is a logical disjunction between symbolic mental functions and the biological brain functions subserving them [1].

If we divorce language from the brain and try to see it as an abstract, disembodied function, we seem to go in circles [2]. If we use biological reductionism to try to side-step the world knot of mind-brain interaction, we deny the mental component of human life. It seems that only a genuinely integrated account of language as a mental function generated by the brain is likely to be successful. This chapter will show that the biocognitive model can account for both aspects of language, the semantic content and the physical act of speech, while avoiding some of the more obvious philosophical traps.

8-3. When Mental States Communicate

Consider a small experiment. A few days after receiving certain instructions, person A walks through a room and sees several items of furniture and a couple of smaller objects. He then enters a second room where person B is waiting.

To declare the start of the experiment, B fixes A with a quizzical look. "Well?" she asks.

"The book is on the table," A announces.

B then takes a book from a shelf and places it on a small table.

"Correct," A agrees, thereby ending the experiment.

The core of this exchange is that A had certain knowledge and communicated it to B. Thus, in this schema, language is about communicating mental states between capable humans. In any act of communication, A has a mental state and wishes to evoke in B a mental state which stands in some direct relationship to A's own mental state. A might wish B to believe that A is happy, or can see a red flower. A may assert that Caesar is dead, that he (A) is rich, or that he is poor when in fact he is not. In general, A might communicate an independently verifiable fact, or something unproven that everybody agrees is a fact, or something he believes is a fact but nobody else does, or something he deliberately made up to resemble a fact, or something about the future which sounds like a fact but which hasn't even happened. He may wish to affect B in a certain way, influencing her behavior, her opinions or her emotions. The limits of language are the limits of human mental states which, in the main, seem to have rather fewer limits than philosophers have traditionally supposed.

From this point of view, the questions a biocognitive theory of language must answer are as follows:

1. What is a mental state, and how does the speaker acquire one?

2. How does the speaker form an intention to communicate his mental state to another person?

3. How is the speaker's mental state converted into the physical act of speech?

4. How are sound waves perceived and converted into a corresponding mental state in the hearer?

A mental state is any private, inner subjective state which comprises part of the individual's continuing, self-aware experience. In this model, mental states are split into two separate but related categories, the experiential and the knowledge-based. Further, there are two aspects to the informational realm, the cognitive contents and the means by which these contents are manipulated, or cognitive analyzers. The informational content is broadly-based, comprising current knowledge, immediately recoverable and dimly recalled memories, and both explicit and implicit information capable of influencing the behavioral output. This information is coded into the brain at the neuronal level. It is manipulated in dedicated neuronal systems to produce decisions which are then manifest as observable behavior (including emotions) but the actual processing of the information by the cognitive analyzer is not open to introspection. Manipulation of the coded information takes place at a sub-neuronal level but does not involve anything other than ordinary, cell-based activity mediated by chemical neurotransmitters. It is central to this model that the mental state is a self-controlling product of cerebral informational processing. The mental state controls the brain, not the other way around. Because the information is coded into neurons which are themselves directly connected to the afferent tracts of the CNS, there is no jump from insubstantial spirit to material body. Rather, the significance of the neuronal impulses depends on where they take place. There is no such thing as disembodied information, nor can information survive the destruction of the physical substrate in which it is encoded.

So, to return to the experiment. Some days before the exchange outlined above, A is recruited and given his instructions. He memorizes them and, on the due date, reports for what sounds like an easy $5.00. That is, he arrives at the outer room with a considerable body of knowledge coded into his brain and available for the experiment. Part of this is the language they speak: he can therefore understand the instruction: "Walk through the room and note where the book is, then tell the researcher in the next room." Without thinking of this explicitly, he sees the book, pushes open the second door (again relying on unstated information of what doors normally do) and recognizes a human being waiting for him. How do we recognize things? We don't, the brain does it for us. So, by completing the task, A acts on his intention to get his money. I do not propose that he arrives at the second room rehearsing in his head his statement to the researcher; rather, he simply looks at B and the words come. Not only do the right words come, but they are in correct order, intonation and everything else we would take for granted about language. But speech should never be taken for granted, it is far too complex.

The hearer, B, perceives certain sounds and immediately appreciates what A means to convey. Before she can do this, the sound waves from A's mouth must be converted into neuronal impulses in B's inner ear, then conveyed to her brain via the acoustic nuclei. The particular patterns of sound evoke certain responses in her brain which, collectively, generate the mental "meaning" of A's sentence. Thus aware, B signals her new knowledge by physical action, which negates the possibility of misunderstanding. This is performed without anything that could be called "conscious awareness." B's comprehension of A's spoken words is so fast as to feel immediate. She does not have to wonder what the sound "book" means, nor scan everything in the room until she finds one. She does not concentrate on her subsequent action nor will it in the sense that a person recovering from a nerve injury has to will his limb to move. The function of language is the evocation of related mental states which then provide the basis for further action.

8-4. How Mental States Evoke Like Mental States

When A arrives at the room, he has coded into his brain a series of instructions able to participate in the hugely complex computational processes which determine his behavior. They are "his" intentions in the respect that he is capable of changing them if he wishes. It is a simple matter of over-riding one behavioral program by another (some behavioral programs, of course, may be acquired implicitly and therefore not be amenable to direct intervention). He walks into the experimental room and glances around. In a matter of milliseconds, coded information has flowed from his retina, through the brainstem nuclei to the primary visual cortex, whence it is relayed to the association cortex. At each point in this process, the informational flow is filtered and modified such that only a highly derivative form reaches the cortex. It then flows through a cascade of highly specific neurons which function as logic gates, meaning they are able to make the elementary decisions into which even the most complex questions can be disassembled. All of this takes place very fast at a level of function which cannot be introspected. From this process arise two quite separate but intimately related matters, first, the experience of seeing something that looks bookish on a flat, wooden surface and, secondly, the knowledge events: "table," "book" and "on." Without deliberating on either mental experience, he passes into the second room and delivers his answer to the researcher.

The question is: *how does this take place?*

The data flow which enters the visual cortex consists of a flow of neuronal impulses. These carry the partially-encoded data from which the actual conscious experience and knowledge (of a book on a table) will be generated. Presumably, data travels from the primary to the secondary cortex and thence to the visual association cortex but the precise details are not yet known and don't matter: once in the cortex, it flows through a complex array of logic gates which process it to the point where conscious experience and knowledge emerge to constitute part of the mental state. A mental state is not a flow of neuronal impulses. It is a higher-order function, an element of a virtual machine which is generated by the manipulation of neuronal data flows by the complex structure of the cerebral cortex. Part of that machine is a series of private, virtual images flickering in and out of existence while the other part is information which can form the basis of behavior and communication. The coded information of the knowledge state is not open to introspection but is directed to effector centers of the brain, including, among others, the limbs, the speech centers and the emotional centers. Knowledge evokes observable output states, although one of the output states, emotion, is only experienced by the subject himself. That is, the sensory input must first be dismantled into its elementary parts until it is of a form which can be processed by the final steps of the recognition process. This takes place in the microstructure of the association cortex, specifically in neurons whose thousands of axonal inputs allow them to function as logic gates. The information is then in a form where it can interact with other information coded in the brain, especially memory traces.

We can assume the recognition process takes the generic form of all such processes, such as:

> If (four legs) and (flat surface) and (surface on top of legs) logically implies (table).

This type of decision-making is ubiquitous in nature. It can be physical, chemical, electrochemical, electronic or even photonic but it always takes the form of elementary logical processes. Critically, these can be mechanized, meaning the highest order mental decisions can be reduced to a lengthy series of primitive steps which can be performed by a mindless machine, be it a human brain or a human artifact. Needless to say, the same principles apply in all brains, not just human. The only difference is the complexity of the cortical cytoarchitecture, which determines the numbers of connections between neurons. On the afferent side, incoming information is dismantled, logical operations are performed on its elemental units, and then the efferent instructions are assembled from these units. In many respects, the principle being developed here is similar to digestion, in which complex chemicals are ingested, digested, absorbed and then reprocessed to manufacture different, complex chemicals in the service of the body.

For a simple action, such as picking up a ball and throwing it, the processes are not difficult to conceptualize. The visual input provokes a recognition of "ball" which in turn recalls an instruction coded in memory, to the effect: "Pick up a ball and throw it back." The memory is coded as synaptic modifications which affect the flow of neuronal impulses, meaning they are in the same form as the data flowing from the association cortex. Thus, the incoming information ("ball") is able to interact directly with the memory traces, based in the same neuronal structure:

If (recognize ball) implies (pick up ball) logically implies (throw ball).

The final decision, "throw the ball," is also in the same coded form as the input and memory, namely synaptic modifications of neuronal impulses. This decision immediately proceeds to the motor organizer [4] and thence to the various subunits of the vast, distributed motor effector system (telencephalic and mesencephalic structures, cerebellum, motor cortex), then down the pyramidal tracts to the anterior horn cells. At no time, from the instant the light rays impact upon the retina to the moment of relaxation of the flexors of the fingers, is there anything like a conscious awareness of these high speed, brain-based processes. I am aware that it is my intention to pick up the ball, but that is a memory function. People forced to make instantaneous decisions often comment on how they didn't think about it, they just acted. Information processing is fast and silent. It has to be fast, otherwise we would never have survived this long, and the only way it can be fast is by bypassing all potential points of delay, of which the major one is the internal theatre of conscious experience. I am reaching for the ball at the instant I see it: our survival as a species depends on the fastest possible responses to the environment, and the fastest possible responses are unthinking or automated responses.

We can now answer the first question: What is a mental state, and how does the speaker acquire one?

There are two sorts of mental states, experiential, and computational, of which only the latter have causative significance. A computational mental state is a cluster of informational states, including current input and explicitly and implicitly acquired memory. Neuronal activity constitutes the physical substrate by which the information is carried, just as pulses of electrical activity in a copper wire, or light impulses in a fiber optic cable, constitute the physical substrate by which the information in a telephone call is carried. When neurons interact at the synaptic junction with the soma, their informational content is altered in predictable ways. Thus, a mental state develops when the current informational input interacts with the individual's near-infinite memory stores to produce a coherent output.

Secondly, how does the speaker form an intention to communicate his mental state to another person?

An intention to speak arises when the interaction of the information in the memory and the current input triggers a cluster of instructions to the speech centers. The process is similar in principle to a thermostat: the furnace is switched on when the memory state (programmed instructions) interacts with the current input (from the temperature gauge) to trigger an instruction to the switch controlling the heating element. In human psychology, however, there are countless factors involved in making even the simplest decision, so many that it may be better to say that the instructions to the speech centers emerge from a "cloud" of instructions and other information in a virtual space. The emergence of a single outcome from the myriad instructions is experienced as an intention to speak.

8-5. How Mental States Evoke Speech

It might be objected that this dehumanizes speech but it points to an overarching principle in this entire project. This is to give an account of language that does not rely on magical entities to complete the causative chain, yet which preserves the essence of humanity, free will and thence, creative speech. As Isaac Bashevis Singer commented: "There must be free will. We have no choice in that." Any account of language must explain the infinite range of human speech without invoking supernatural spirits (e.g. the magical Self of Popper and Eccles [5]) which lead to an infinite regress [1] and are therefore non-scientific. Thus, given a sufficiently large number of memories (including hopes, aims, goals, likes and dislikes, etc.) interacting with the endlessly-changing current sensory input, the language output is essentially infinite. However, each of these language elements is mindless, so there is no "tiny mind" directing them, just their own logic. On this basis, the vast complexity of human speech is assembled from mindless elements. However, this is emphatically not the same as Kandel's claim that birdsong and human speech can be explained by the same elementary biological processes. There are layers upon layers of complexity between the simple, repetitive elements of a bird's mating call and the infinite creativity of human speech. Physiologically, the bird brain lacks the neuronal elements I have called logic gates, meaning it is not capable of analyzing incoming data to the extent of a human brain. Birds emit characteristic, repetitive calls because that is all they are capable of perceiving. Anything more complex is lost as their brains lack the computational power to understand the semantic significance of "Polly want a cracker?"

An answer to the next question, of how the speaker's mental state is converted into the physical act of speech, depends precisely upon a conceptual resolution of the mind-body problem. Chapters 4-6 argue that the point of contact between the virtual realm of the mind and its physical substrate is where the informational content of a nerve impulse acts to influence another nerve cell body, such that it either facilitates or blocks transmission in the second nerve. That is, contiguous neurons act as logic gates to the informational content their impulses carry. Thus, an assembly of closely-associated neurons process the cloud of information to the point where there is a particular outcome. Physically, this consists of an array of impulses in dedicated neurons, probably located in the prefrontal cortex. These instructions then activate the next step in the process, ordinary conductive neurons which transmit the output to the first stages of the speech centers. It should be understood that there is a very important difference in function between neurons which are interconnected such that they can function as logic gates, and "mere" conductive neurons which transmit instructions from one part of the brain to the next but do not process them. These functional differences are real, despite the vital point that all neuronal action potentials are exactly the same. The real activity depends on how the neurons are wired together, as it were, and whether they form excitatory or inhibitory junctions. This is where the brain's many neurotransmitters become important: it is perfectly feasible for a single neuron to utilize different transmitters depending on where its axons are directed.

So impulses in one section of the brain are processed as data, then shipped out to the next step in the distributed process called "making a decision." There is no reason why this should not be repeated a dozen times or more between the retina and the lips, where each relay processes the data further and sends it forward to the next step. The final outcome, a well-formed sentence, is a direct product of the mental state that preceded it. In the materialist ethos, summarized by the slogan, "Everything has a real cause," the cause of a sentence just is its preceding mental state. That is, a sentence does not stand in a necessary relationship of truth or falsity with the real world, it simply reflects what the subject believed as he uttered the words, and a person can believe anything. If a sentence does in fact stand in a truthful relationship to the real world, that is a contingent fact, not necessary.

To return to our experiment: A leaves the first room with several concepts in his head, where the expression "in his head" is used advisedly, as the concepts are entirely virtual. These can include: Get $5.00, on, book, enter second room, buy beer, notify experimenter, table. At this stage, we don't need to explain precisely how the different behavioral elements (enter second room, buy beer, notify experimenter) interact as that is conceptually not difficult, and chimps can sequence their behavior anyway (one renowned student of chimp behavior even observed them using deception to capture another animal, [6]). What is of interest here is how a speech act is assembled. To explain this, it will be necessary to digress a little.

Analyzing, or parsing, a sentence reduces it to its constituent parts until they can be seen in relation to each other. Take a simple sentence: The boy is eating some cake.

This is parsed as: The (definite article or determiner) boy (subject noun) is eating (verb/present continuous tense) some (partitive article) cake (object noun).

Diagrammatically, this is shown on Fig. 8-1 (following page)

In Indonesian, the same event would be described as: *Anak makan kue.* In Bahasa Indonesia, there are no articles and no tenses, yet the hearer will understand the same meaning as an English speaker hearing the first sentence. That is, each sentence expresses the same three concepts, and concepts are irreducibly mental states. All the other parts of the sentence are added without conscious intent by a native speaker, and amount to the difference between somebody who can see the boy but cannot express it in a particular tongue, compared with somebody who "speaks the language." It is the case that a person watching the boy does not see articles and tenses. Observing him yields three concepts: "boy," "cake," and "cake disappearing

```
                    ┌─────────────────────────────────┐
                    │   The boy is eating some cake.  │
                    └─────────────────────────────────┘
```

The boy is eating some cake.

Noun phrase (subject):

Verb phrase: is eating some

Definite article: The

Noun: boy

Verb: is eating

Noun phrase (object):

Partitive article: some

Noun: cake.

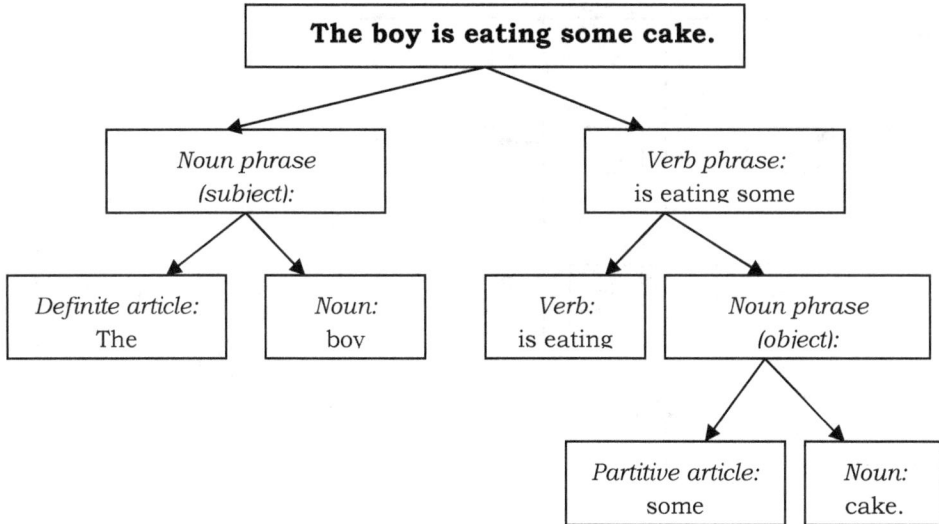

Fig. 8-1: Diagramming a sentence

into boy." These three concepts amount to two things and one relationship between the two things. For communication to occur, they must be assembled into a coherent structure such that a listener can extract the information which the speaker intends to convey. Just as German speakers "unconsciously" place the verbs at the end of their sentence in reverse order, so English speakers insert all sorts of qualifiers in their sentences without thinking about them.

I suggest this does not happen in the same section of the brain as subserves concept manipulation, but in lower-order speech centers. That is, the concepts are manipulated until they stand in correct relationship (The boy ate the cake, not *vice versa*) and only then are these items sent to a center where articles, etc. are added. Subsequently, the whole bundle of instructions is sent to the motor centers governing the actual physical act of speech. Effectively, this is parsing in reverse order. A native speaker constructs a sentence from its elements and the hearer deconstructs it to extract just those elements, i.e. to discover its meaning. The meaning of a sentence just is the elements the speaker wishes to convey.

If we modify the parsing diagram in Fig. 8-1 so that it shows a time span along the x-axis and space along the y-axis, we arrive at a diagram of an assembly line for sentences, as it were (see Fig. 8-2):

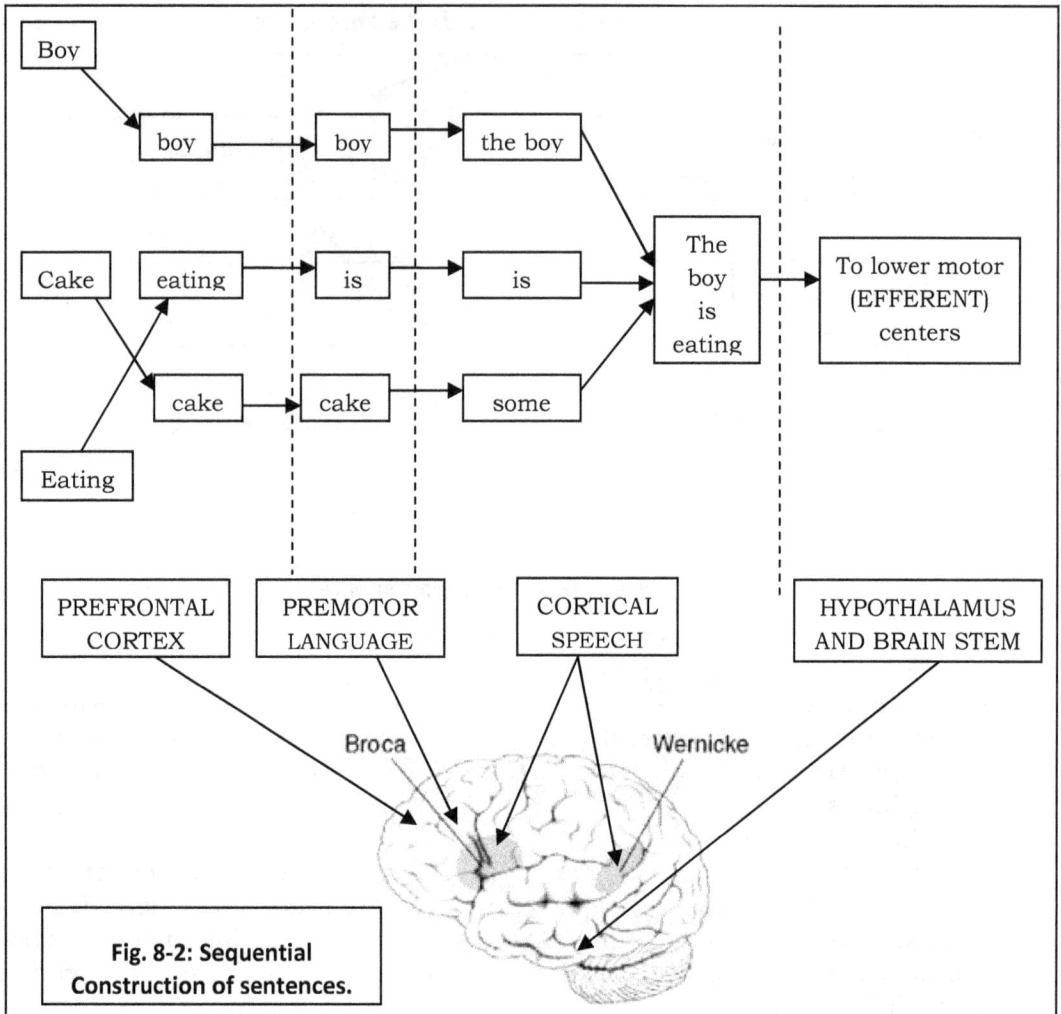

Fig. 8-2: Sequential Construction of sentences.

In this model, the starting point of any utterance is a mental state consisting of certain items of information which the speaker wishes to convey to his audience. Metaphorically, these items are floating in a conceptual space in the head where they can interact with instructions coded in memory. In the experiment, the items (get $5.00, on, book, enter second room, buy beer, notify experimenter, table) interact with the memorized instruction: "To get the money, tell the experimenter where the book is." As a result, the information is directed to the preliminary language centers (possibly equivalent to Luria's language organizer). By a series of steps which do not involve conscious intent but rely on memorized rules alone, the concepts are ordered according to the grammar of that particular language; articles and other qualifiers are added, then the final message is dispatched to the neurological speech centers.

This approach disassembles the generation of language into a series of perfectly rational steps, starting with the mental concepts and then organizing them into a rule-governed sequence. There seems little doubt that the different steps actually take place in different parts of the brain, starting with the prefrontal cortex and ending in the brainstem centers that control the diaphragm and the muscles of the larynx. This is a highly complex process but it is conceptually simple. It can be interrupted at any of perhaps dozens of points, producing the well-known disturbances of speech seen in neurology.

The process of assembling a sentence is very fast. Native speakers do not have time to consider, in any real sense of the term, the exact order and intonation of what they are about to say. At the time of initiating an utterance, we have a notion of just what to say, i.e. a cluster of ideas, but the exact form of the sentence that will carry just that notion to the hearer emerges as the sentence unfolds. The brain does all that for us. Sentences are assembled from constituent elements just as a car is assembled in a factory: the elements are arranged in order as they move along a predetermined path, and then other bits are added until the finished product pops out at the other end. When speaking, I do not know the third next word I will use, but it will be correct in grammar and intonation, perhaps surprising even me with its perspicacity—or its clumsiness.

8-7. How Speech Evokes Mental States

The speaker's larynx, lips, tongue and teeth combine to produce particular sounds which convey meaning, but only to someone who knows the particular code or language. Everybody can hear, but only native speakers understand the language, meaning they can decode the sounds to form the mental state the speaker intended for them. The patterns of rapid variations in air pressure which are generated by the speaker are detected by the hearer's ear, a remarkably sensitive organ which, if it were any more sensitive, would be able to detect the Brownian movement of air molecules. The physiology of the ear is such that it amplifies soft sounds and dampens loud, meaning it is effective across a vast range of volumes, from a faint whisper to the sound of thunder directly overhead. Because it can detect many different frequencies at the same time, the ear provides the basis for selective hearing, which is essential for survival. When a sound impinges on the tympanic membrane, it provokes a series of neuronal impulses in the acoustic nerve which carry the coded information to the brain. Similar to the visual system, the barrage of impulses passes through a series of brainstem nuclei where the pattern is manipulated before it arrives at the auditory cortex. Here, it is further analyzed by passing through arrays of logic gates until it yields its significance (usually known as meaning).

Once again, the incoming information is somehow split in two parts, one part forming the basis of the experience of hearing a sound and the other part providing information on which actions are based. In our experiment, the speaker says: "The book is on the table." From this, the hearer gains information which constitutes a mental state standing in a precise relationship with the speaker's mental state, namely, that something with pages is located on the upper part of a flat surface supported by four legs. Specifically, she apprehends that there is a table and there is a book, and the table is under the book. She doesn't actually have to think about this, the information is derived from the neuronal data flow as it filters through the analyzers of the auditory association cortex and becomes part of her instantaneous mental state or consciousness. But what is an analyzer? Is it just a bit of hip jargon used to conceal a sly little homunculus, a sort of Mechanical Turk bridging the gap between brain and mind? We have to be very careful about these types of terms as they need to be explained in detail. We have to ensure that, not only are there no explanatory gaps which need to be filled but there are no possible points at which miraculous interventions could occur.

I don't know what an analyzer looks like. I presume it is a complex of neurons (similar to the classic picture of cortical histology) which functions as an array of on-off switches to break incoming data streams into recognizable components and then using these to trigger information coded in memory. So, the sound conveyed by these marks "table" activates a cluster of memories of flat surfaces supported on four legs; the sound of the word "book" brings up a range of memories of thick wads of printed paper, and the sound of "on" brings the first cluster of memories into a particular relationship with the second cluster. That is, the sound waves generated by the speaker using the code known as English evoke a fleeting mental state in the hearer just because she can decode those sounds, and the process of decoding builds in her mind a very accurate reflection or version of what was in the speaker's mind. The whole point of a spoken language is to create in the hearer's mind a facsimile of the speaker's mental state. Of course, this is also true of written and other languages.

Entities, including humans, "talk" to each other using codes to convey information. Sometimes the information works directly, such as using a card to open a gate. In humans, the purpose may be solely to convey factual infor-mation as in this example, other times the total mental state the speaker wishes to convey can include his ambition to provoke certain emotional responses in his audience. A language is thus the vehicle by which mental states are communicated. Mental states are evoked not just by factual information (which may or may not be correct) but also a range of emotional triggers ("Look out!"), instructions ("Stand still, laddy!"), claims about the future ("Now for the weather forecast"), fiction and fantasy, deceptions ("Of course I'll respect you in the morning"), exclamations of various types ("Yuck!" and anything that rhymes with it), fillers and social clutter ("Charmed, I'm sure"), songs, and various other non-verbal conduits of information about the speaker's mental state. Any system of codes which conveys one person's mental state to another (or, for machines, one informational state to another) is called a language. Languages convey information about the immaterial realm in one entity (called the mind in humans) across the void to another, receptive entity. Conveying truth is only a small part of what humans do with their marvelous faculty called language.

I think one of the biggest problems in talking about language is that we take this fantastically complex process for granted. When two native speakers converse, it all seems so effortless that we don't give it a moment's thought. But if speech were so simple, somebody should explain why only humans have the gift and why computers can't write novels.

8-8. Summary of the Model

Figure 8-3 shows some of the relationships between different uses and modes of language but I am sure the reality of language is much more complex than this. This is a decision tree, which subdivides all forms of communication according to their functional status. In this respect, it differs from most other approaches, which tend to be concerned with, for example, truth properties. This is first and last a psychological analysis of language. It proposes that sentences are assembled sequentially from their elements by an orderly process (i.e. it takes time) involving centers located in different parts of the brain substance. That is, sentences do not "arrive in consciousness" as complete entities but are built from smaller elements which, by themselves, have no "meaning." Meaning, as we use the word, emerges from the cloud of meaningless elements, just as a cake emerges from a cluster of non-cake elements (it is a cloud if you try to count each individual grain of flour). The meaning of a sentence is not a magical process conjured into existence by a clever little man hidden in the head. It is a perfectly rational matter of two sentient beings using an agreed code to match their informational states by a series of real, coherent processes that are beyond introspection.

On the speaker's side, the crucial elements of a sentence are the separate items of information he wishes to impart. The actual word order of the resulting sentence involves a number of mechanical processes *outside introspective range* which assemble the items in the correct order for that language, then decorate them with the little bits that convert it from a crude pidgin or Creole to the fully-developed language. Only the first part of this process involves the mind as we normally use the term: "To my mind, you drive too fast." The rest is simple mechanics, as it were, automated industrial robots that add bits to the sentence, rearrange it, polish it and then speed the instructions on their way to the emitters (larynx, etc.). It should not be forgotten that even the simplest speech act involves a massive effort of coordination at the neurological level. For example, people with certain sorts of brain damage lose the capacity to coordinate their diaphragmatic action with the inner rhythm of the sentence. As a result, the verbal emphasis in the sentence is wrong, and they may run out of breath mid-sentence. All of this takes place outside the realm of what people call consciousness, in that it is very fast and cannot be introspected. That does not, however, imply that it is not intentional. When I decide to do something, I simply send the instructions to the relevant centers and they do the rest. Agreed, learning to type or play the piano or drive are more difficult processes, but once those behavioral programs are committed to motor memory, they involve no more intention than, say, following a letter through the post office after I have posted it. I trust the system will do its duty.

On the hearer's side, the process is reversed. In the natural economy of neurological systems, it would make sense to use the same brain systems where possible but simply to reverse their activity. This generalization needs to be investigated empirically but, at a system level, it is of value in understanding the twin processes of language generation and language comprehension. The generative process assembles sentences out of mental concepts while the comprehension process unpacks those sentences to get at the mental concepts or meaning that they carry. There is nothing difficult about the essential notion involved: if I told you that this factory assembles washing machines from parts gathered from all over the country, even the world, while the factory across the road dismantles them when they have reached the end of their lifespan (about six months, these days), and recycles the bits, then you wouldn't think twice about it. You would not see it as mysterious or forever beyond human ken, you would not need to imagine clever little demons hidden inside the automated welding machines. This is also true of the brain when it acquits that quintessentially human activity called talking to each other. While it is vastly (but probably not immeasurably) complex, the basic processes are, well, basic. At our present level of knowledge, we just have a little problem with the actual codes the brain uses but that is not essential: I can work with MS-Windows without ever knowing their proprietary machine code.

It must not be forgotten that this is a theory of language. That is, it is my offering to shed light on the unseen mechanisms which are interposed between hearing a sentence and responding. It is a proposal of how the brain does its job which, I hope, does not beg any questions, invoke any unprovable entities, or involve small miracles ("But daddy, it's just a very *small* puppy...."). By "unseen mechanisms," I mean not only the actual neurological structures but, more importantly, the coded rules that drive those structures to do what they do. It must not be forgotten that language is a rule-driven process. Granted, a crucial feature of any language is its astounding creativity but language itself is not the creative process, it is merely one of the vehicles of that creativity. Creativity is a mental phenomenon, not a language phenomenon, any more than a CD is a part of the creative process for a musician. The endless variety of a spoken language is the result of the myriad of informational states that impel it, and that is why I used the term "cloud." I believe we may never know exactly what information the brain uses to construct even a simple sentence. Even if I say exactly the same sentence every day of my life, it will never quite be the same, subtle changes of intonation will intrude and these have meaning somewhere. Whether that meaning amounts to anything is moot; the biocognitive model does not claim, as psychoanalysis did, that every mistake is not a mistake. I can stumble over my speech just because, very briefly, another thought intruded or because I am most anxious that you do not doubt what I am saying.

8-9. Scope of the Model

8-9 (a). Thought disorder

With this distributed account of communication (i.e. neurology of speech plus semantics of language), the biocognitive model satisfies common observation yet avoids an infinite regress and leaves room for creativity (via free will). It immediately provides a rational basis for the disturbances of speech first charted by Broca and by Westphal. More significantly for psychiatry, because the model involves the notion of mental states (including rules) as the primary determinants of language, we can account for the thought disorders of the major psychiatric syndromes without invoking an impairment of the brain's organic state. This model generates an account of thought disorder from first principles: mental disorder does not imply brain disorder [1]. In the case of the garbled language seen in mental disorder, the basic principle is quite simple: for whatever reason, the thought-disordered person's set of linguistic rules is malfunctioning. This might be due to over-arousal, or a powerful need to hide something, or just that, from years of distress, the standard rules of language have lost their significance because they no longer accurately convey the suffering person's mental state. Thus, he twists the rules of language in his attempts to convey what is important to him (and sometimes to conceal what is important). Look at the following examples of an intelligent and introspective man with a ten year history of mental disorder:

My Schizophrenia

I measure a being in the reflection of words that has no measure, no beginning and no end—parallel of the comparative life that is a mere naming of shadows, i.e. measure the word tall.

It is of returning from the created into creation, leaving the measure of time, life and death—the shadows of paranoia, and passing into existence.

My ignorance is my measure.

A Dimension of Delusion

As viewed from a spatial dimension in a corner of my mind, a picture at a wall of a room appears as a pattern of a tiger-skin in a defined pose of a kangaroo.

Which is it, and how do I know that it has not the heart of a lamb or a potato, and what does it matter? I must be drunk in a measure of ignorance for the skin or cast of a thing, which blinds me of its essence, and in this state of mentality I can only judge a thing in a cast of my definitions.

Habit is of ignorance and both are of delusion. How shall I loosen the ignorance of my measure when there is no measure of ignorance? What is in a name other than an existence?

Och, oi! What a funny planet, every creature ignorant in its delusions. When shall I cease to be a fool, and is such a thing possible in ignorance?

I Don't Know It's All Delusional

The light of truth and the moon of learning—ignorance and delusion the order of the day, but in a delusion of ignorance where defining ceases there is only existence; but I don't know, I can't make sense—it ceases with defining, I can only exist and be delusional; but really I don't know, nor can I pretend. As a blind man once said, "we live in ignorance as we die." There is no god only God.

The young man's strain of trying to convey something terribly important is manifest. If he could control it a little better, people would acclaim him as a poet.

From the theoretical point of view, the biocognitive model can easily account for thought disorder just by proposing that the normal rules of language (governing what will be said and in what order) have failed for some reason and the individual is no longer using the words of the language in the same way as everybody else, no longer following the rules of the code. This is, I believe, a far more parsimonious and probable explanation than the organic model, which proposes that the actual physical centers subserving language are subtly damaged when nothing else is. The biological model doesn't include rules: it has no place for rules just because rules are not biological in nature, they are immaterial.

8-9 (b). Knowledge and the biocognitive model

At this stage of the development of the biocognitive model, it is probably a bit presumptuous to outline a theory of knowledge but that is all it will be, an outline. Theories of knowledge, or epistemology, are an integral part of the Western intellectual tradition. Attempts to analyze what we know, what we can know, how we know that what we believe is reliable, etc., go back to the earliest Greek writings: "The starting point in analyzing the concept of knowledge—determining what knowledge is—is to ask what knowledge is *not*" [7; his emphasis]. Traditional views of knowledge excluded ignorance, error and opinion [8] but the model of language developed above does not sit easily with this very restrictive view. The biocognitive approach is that language is driven by mental states, and mental states have many purposes, hence language is much broader than merely the vehicle of truth (or error, or opinion, etc.). A theory of epistemology then becomes a theory of mental states, meaning epistemology is an aspect of an overarching theory of mind, which is what the biocognitive model hopes to be.

Looking again at Fig. 8-3, it is clear that communication takes many forms (vocal, written, signs, portents, etc). Vocal communication itself divides into linguistic (using words) and non-linguistic, meaning yells, laughter and various grunts, sighs and wailings in between. Non-linguistic vocalizations communicate something about the utterer's mental state to a person within earshot. Most of these are driven by the innate cognitive system, meaning they are better at communicating emotional states than factual knowledge. Within linguistic forms of communication, we can readily differentiate between formed sentences and unformed sentences. The latter include various greetings and salutations which serve the role of social lubricants but don't convey much factual information ("Good morning." "My dear, you're looking so well." "You're so kind. Have a nice day." "And what did she mean by that?"). Similar kinds of interchanges involving obscenity and other idioms can be heard every day in the street or workplace.

Formed sentences can express propositions but, at least as commonly, they do not. Examples of non-propositional formed sentences include orders and commands ("Company, stand at ease!" "OK, driver, let me see your license" "I'd like you to close the door."). These convey something important about the utterer's mental state which the hearer would be ill-advised to ignore. They do not express anything that can be considered truthful in any meaningful sense of the word but the world would soon grind to a halt if we didn't have this ability. There are other classes of non-propositional formed sentences, including emotional ventings ("I'd like a dollar for every time I've told you not to do that." "Goodness me, what a fuss"), ceremonial declarations ("I hereby declare you man and wife." "This honorable court is now in session."), direct questions ("Tell the court, did you or did you not hit him?"), rhetorical questions which don't demand an answer ("I ask you, what sort of fool are you?" "Having a bad day, are we?"), various figures of speech and allegory ("The market dived today as punters got a haircut and black gold tanked but King Midas blossomed late so early toe-cutters were hosed down") and so on.

The question is not whether any of this is true in any stringent sense of the word but whether the speaker can convey his particular mental state to his intended audience. That is all that counts. Attempts to assign truth values to non-propositional formed sentences simply tie the author in knots. It is important not to lose sight of common sense: "Truth is the most valuable thing we have. Let us economize it" (Mark Twain).

Propositional formed sentences are sentences with a declarative content. This can be true, false or something in between but we have to be careful not to beg the question of truth. Some statements appear to express a proposition but they are misleading, e.g. claims about the future. There is no correlation between a statement now and an event which has not happened to which we can assign a meaningful truth value:

> "The sun will rise tomorrow."
> "I say you're wrong."
> "And I say it's true."
> "What, that you believe it or that it will rise?"
> "Both."
> "Then prove it. If your claim is true now, then you must have proof now."

There are many, many mental states we can convey to another person in the form of a valid proposition but which have no parallel in the real world. All fiction falls into this class even though it may express something reliable: "It is true that the penguins hijacked a ship to sail to Antarctica" means only: "Within the fictional world of the film, *Madagascar*, it is true that the penguins hijacked a ship to sail to Antarctica." It also happens that we may try to say something truthful but the form of the sentence is such that it permits the hearer to form two differing mental states rather than one, i.e. the sentence is ambiguous. One or other interpretation of an ambiguous sentence may be true but the test of any expression is not what the speaker intends but what the hearer discerns. Nonsensical sentences do not convey anything just because the words cannot be used together, giving a failure of reference: "Colorless green ideas sleep furiously" (Chomsky's example). A lot of political speeches fit this category, but rarely by accident.

This has narrowed the field of human utterances considerably; all that remain are formed sentences which express a proposition that can rightly be classified as truthful. Once again, we can divide them in two groups, those expressing universal truths, including truism and mathematics, and those expressing specific truths, including empirical truth and metaphysical truth. Mathematics is an interesting category, as it expresses relationships which are necessarily true: 1+1=2 is true just because it could not be otherwise. Pythagoras' theorem is true just because that is the nature of a right-angled triangle, and not because there is anything magical about it. As a result, many people would say that mathematics doesn't have anything to do with a theory of knowledge. Progress in mathematics is just progress in uncovering relationships that have existed since the beginning of time; the only value of knowing the relationships is that they might allow us to predict future events more precisely: "Here's to pure mathematics," as the toast goes, "may it never be of use to anybody."

I have lumped together historical and scientific truth or empirical truth with matters that are true by definition, such as law, ethical systems and so on. Because this is a materialist ontology, there is no place for received truth. Religious truth becomes a matter of definition by the group involved: is it true that the world was made in just seven days? Yes, if you accept a particular view of the universe but not otherwise. Is it true that drivers caught speeding must pay a fine? Yes, in that jurisdiction; in others, they simply pay a bribe and speed off. Truth inheres in mental states; language is just the vehicle of that mental state as it is conveyed to the hearer.

Some statements can be shown to be true as a matter of definition. They are analytically true, meaning their truth can be demonstrated by an analysis of the meaning of the words involved. They are not empirical truths, because they cannot be refuted by experience. There is, for example, no fact or observation which could change the meaning of the word "speeding" as defined in the traffic code. Synthetic statements assert facts whose truth can only be verified by referring back to the world of facts. An analytic truth can masquerade as a synthetic truth but not vice versa.

8-9 (c). Epistemological consequences of the biocognitive model

Sentences do not refer forward to the world; any truth in the relationship of a sentence to the real world is contingent, not necessary. It is pointless to attempt to establish the "truth" of a sentence independently of the mental state that evoked it. A mental state stands in a precise relationship with the sentence it generates, even if the sentence is a lie. The reference point of any sentence is its originating mental state, not the real world. A sentence refers back to its originating mental state in much the same sense as a sausage refers back to the sausage machine that made it. Sausages are innocent of truth and obscenity; they are victims of the sausage machine. A sentence is the "dumb servant" of its originating mental state.

Establishing the truth of a mental state is such a slippery notion that I see very little point in attempting to define the conditions under which we could say: "Her mental state is true." For example, she may say she sees a red rose. We accept that her sentence refers back to her conscious experience, but is it true that what she sees exists in the world? Most definitely not. There are no colors in a world without eyes: colors are generated in a private virtual space only when light of a certain wavelength impinges upon appropriate receptors suitably connected to a highly efficient data processing system. Without eyes, there is no morning sunlight, only electromagnetic energy bathing the chloroplasts. Try telling a worm that it is true there is a rainbow overhead (that's right: no head).

Our mental states are an approximation of the world that exists independently of our crude senses. What we apprehend is "good enough" to survive, meaning it is a pretty good approximation of "out there," but it is only an approximation. What we see of the world, including our neighbors, is what we need to survive. We err on the side of caution because our bolder ancestors who didn't soon met a sticky end. We are able to see in a particular part of the EM spectrum just because it gives us the maximum information about "out there" with the least biological effort. Eyes are a very efficient way of working out where the danger lies, that's why they have evolved about seventeen times. Cats don't have color vision so they can't tell red from brown; they can't tell a poppy from a cowpat because they can't eat poppies and cowpats can't eat them. Instead, they have monochrome vision with a posterior retinal reflector which amplifies the light falling on their on-off receptors where we would have crowded color receptors. This gives them a remarkably acute awareness of movement in low light conditions, i.e. night vision.

The hearer understands the speaker if and only if the hearer's evoked mental state stands in a direct relationship to the originating mental state in the speaker, namely, it is precisely the relationship the speaker intended her to gain. Since there is so much information in the "cloud" from which an intention to speak gels, it is most unlikely that, except in highly artificial circumstances, the hearer's mental state will be more than an approximation of the speaker's mental state, but that is "good enough." Anything more would take too much energy and would become inefficient. Everything has a cause, and this includes every sentence, but we are not able to introspect all the causes. A speaker can't be sure of setting up a facsimile of his mental state in the hearer, just because the speaker isn't aware himself of all that went into his sentence. He may have to correct himself when it emerges. A speaker does not describe his mental state; rather, his instantaneous mental state computes an instruction to speak from current information, memory, etc. It is true to say that the speaker just is his mental state at that moment. Similarly, a sentence spoken without an audience is meaningless noise; the meaning of a sentence just is the mental state it evokes, and if it doesn't evoke one, then it is meaningless. There is no language act without a simultaneous hearing act because communication involves two people. However, I can still talk to myself because I have a memory.

Compare this with Schopenhauer's Principle of Sufficient Reason: Nothing is without a reason. This is not the same as Baruch Spinoza's doctrine: "There is no such thing as Freewill. The mind is induced to wish this or that by some cause, and that cause is determined by another cause, and so on back to infinity." On a simplistic reading, this would lead to the absurd position where, if we went back far enough in time, every event today would have had the same originating event. The more sophisticated approach is that everything has a final cause, but there are myriad factors which lead to that particular outcome and, if things had been ever so slightly different, the outcome may have been the same or it could have been profoundly different. If the infant Hitler had succumbed to whooping cough, would World War II have happened? Maybe, maybe not. But there is free will: I can always examine my habitual responses and improve them if I wish. Trouble is, I think they are already an improvement over my neighbor's habits.

Given all the potential meanings of a sentence, how does the hearer choose the correct one to match the speaker's intent? Even while the speaker is still talking, the listener is restricting the possibilities. We rapidly cull an enormous amount of information, often deciding even before the sentence is finished that it doesn't amount to much; the first few words of a sentence allow us to look ahead and decide whether we need to pay much attention to it. This is second nature: the mind races ahead without any bidding. It is like a footballer or tennis player deciding on the run not to retrieve a shot because it is going to land outside the pitch. If we didn't have the capacity to predict the likely outcome of a particular sentence, we wouldn't be able to laugh at jokes. That is the difference between a child laughing at somebody in a mask saying "boo" and an adult laughing at a sophisticated political joke.

This model seems to have two conflicting aims: to give a materialist account of mind, but also to account for speech by means of mindless processes assembling meaning from meaningless elements. I have repeatedly said it is necessary to ensure that there are no hidden homunculi in the chain of explanation from stimulus to response and back again. That is, every mental process must be given a rational account and cannot be left to emerge from inner space as by magic. The concept of a Self as drawn by Eccles is pure magical thinking. He assigned the essential human features of decision-making etc. to a supernatural entity for which there never could be a rational explanation: it was not a rational or material thing, and could not be held to account in material terms. With respect to a great scientist, his story was mere pseudoscience. Our goal is show how each and every action by a human being can be shown to be the outcome of preceding, rational causes, and language is no different. So, instead of having a creature halfway between angels and animals that generates speech from its supernatural soul, we have to show how the brain can generate speech without the intervention of an obliging soul.

In fact, simply generating speech is the easy bit. We can easily devise programs for desktop computers that will generate speech by algorithm:

> If (time = morning) and (perceive man approaching) and (recognize man) and (wish to be polite to oncoming man) then (speak: "Good morning").

Note that we do not say: "Morn goodning" or "Piss off." Years ago, we learned what will be seen as polite and what won't.

We can easily account for a routine sentence self-constructing from various streams of data flowing through the different neuronal pathways. Elements from the available libraries (memory) click into place until the instruction of what to say and how to say it is sent to the motor centers. By multiplying the streams of data and extending the library so that there are huge numbers of standing instructions on how to speak and what to say interacting with vast streams of data from current perception, memory, etc., we can account for novelty. Machines do this all the time; the difficult bit is accounting for how we zero in on solutions to problems, how we select just one answer from all the possible responses. That is a matter of programming. We can rapidly solve problems by selecting the correct response from a range of options, but only if we restrict the options by limiting the informational input and weighting the parameters correctly. We call that experience. Listen to an experienced politician talking: it sounds impressive but it is only last year's recycled platitudes, an effortless stringing together of trite clichés like sausages strung together—and about as informative. However, it is a different story when you ask him to solve a complex problem. He will refer it to a committee. He may still be remarkably good at discerning the centers of power and finding ways of insinuating himself in them but that is reactive; when it comes to generating true novelty, he has long since suppressed that faculty. He can still recognize it, of course, but it frightens him.

8-9 (d). Moral consequences of the biocognitive model

A materialist account of mind means everything that exists in whatever form has a rational explanation in the real world. It doesn't mean: "Nothing mental in the head" because mentality and materialism are not incompatible. I use the word mental to mean everything that occurs in the informational realm in the head, including conscious experience and the cognitive or knowledge-based functions. A materialist account of language means finding the informational causes of language (as distinct from assigning them to supernatural spirits). A theory of language flows from a theory of mind and, in turn, generates a theory of knowledge (see Fig. 7-1 on p. 103). Everything has a cause, nothing exists in isolation. This allows us to account for morality as an essential feature of human life: in a rule-governed creature, morality just is defined rules. While giving a materialist account of mind, we still need to preserve the notion of the human as a moral actor. It is not contradictory to say that morality exists in a materialist world, but a materialist does not pretend morality is found on mountain tops carved on tablets of stone. There is moral truth, but it is analytically true, like Sherlock Holmes' address.

There are two concepts at work: the idea of a moral system and the idea of a moral actor within that system. Morality is simply a set of rules. We would like those rules to have a purpose but, all too often, the purpose has been lost and the rules have acquired a force of their own ("The Sabbath exists for man..."). For the individual, morality is a simple matter of following rules, something humans do very well. We follow rules well (or should do) because we soak them up from the social and natural environment from infancy. It is a case of learning the rules and abiding by them. However, every decision is the instantaneous outcome of myriad pre-existing factors, so certain rules have to be weighted to the point where they will over-rule most other factors. We have so many rules governing morality but they are computed in exactly the same way as all other rules are computed to generate behavior. All too often, they are contradictory. Homicide is a sin except when the government says it is not.

8-10. Conclusion

The materialist model of mind derived in the earlier chapters of this book can give a productive account of language, and thence a system of knowledge. It avoids concepts such as Forms existing in some other realm or the notion of propositions which exist independently of the sentences that convey them. This model focuses on language as the vehicle of communication of intent; without two people, the speaker and hearer, language loses its role, just as a balloon loses its role if it has no air in it or no air to support it. Language is a code for the communication of mental states; creatures with restricted mental states don't have much to communicate. Unless both parties have learned the code, there is no communication of meaning.

The process of deciding to speak is not much different from the process of deciding to stand up; the brain has a wealth of coded information and some elements of this are used to compute a decision. We cannot introspect the act of making a decision because as soon as the elements come together, there is a decision and it will automatically be sent to the correct effectors. In some neurological diseases, this doesn't happen, which is terribly distressing to the sufferer.

A theory of language which does not proceed from a theory of mind has no anchors in reality and will fly into the void, or become bogged down in pseudo-problems which would not arise if the correct model were in use. The larger model of mind dictates the form of a theory of language, and how it will fit with other areas of human mental activity. For example, the endless fascination for philosophers of language with assigning a role for something called Truth fades when we realize the critical factor in any communication is the originating mental state.

No other model of mind in use in psychiatry today can give an account of language. For this reason alone, the biocognitive model stands in a strong position.

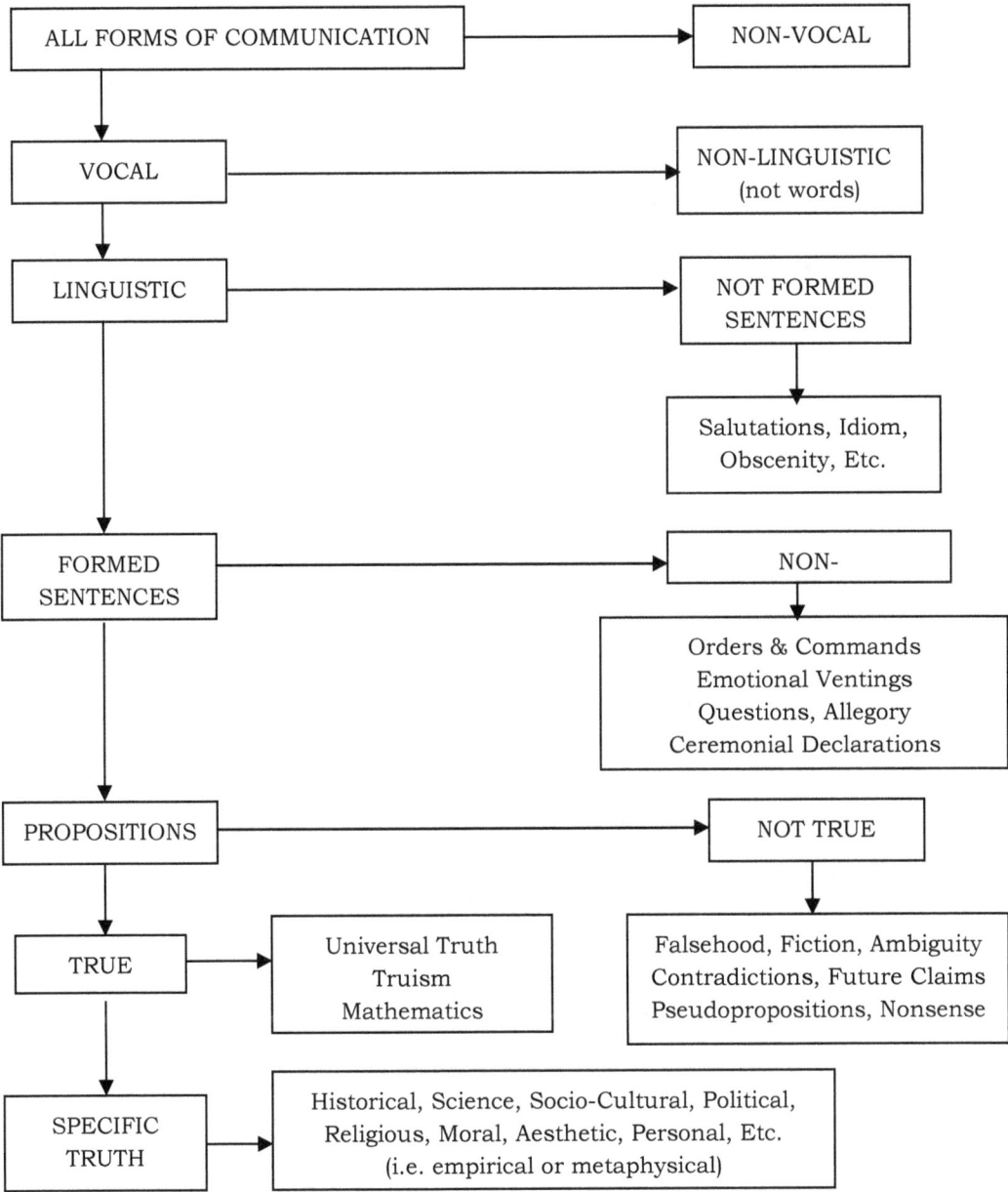

Fig. 8-3: Language array.

9 The Biocognitive Model and Human Nature

"Ghosts:.. There is one insuperable obstacle to a belief in ghosts: a ghost never comes naked... And why does not the apparition of a suit of clothes sometimes walk around without a ghost in it?"
Ambrose Bierce

9-1. Introduction

Because of the importance of a concept of human nature in psychiatry, it is worth reiterating the basic principles on which this theory is assembled so that we don't lose sight of them. I will follow Leslie Stevenson's admirably parsimonious approach to the question.

9-2. A Materialist Reality

9-2 (a). A theory of the world

The ontological stance in this work is the doctrine of materialism, that there is nothing in the universe beyond matter and energy and the informational states controlling them. This approach does not deny the existence of the supernatural realm but insists that it plays no part in the explanation of things. That most astute of observers, Ambrose Bierce, defined prayer as "A plea that the laws of the universe be temporarily annulled in favor of a single petitioner, confessedly unworthy." His point is that there are laws of the universe and they are universal. There is no room for entities, however well-meaning, that are relieved of their duties under, say, the laws of gravity or the inverse-square law. Science proceeds on the basis of regularities; singularities are an affront. However, because materialism provides no means for a rationalist to come to grips with the supernatural, it does not mean it does not exist, only that the rationalist is forever agnostic. She cannot know, just because her fundamental beliefs of the nature of the universe allow her no means of giving an account of the supernatural. That's what "universal laws of nature" means: inviolable, no exceptions.

A materialist stance means that the "natural philosopher" (a most apposite term) has no intellectual or physical means for dealing with the supernatural. This lack of intellectual tools derives from the universality of the laws we discern as fundamental. These are not laws in the sense of something we define ourselves, but they are relationships that exist just because of the physical nature of the universe. It is a law of nature that heat flows from hot things to cold, just because that is the nature of heat, which in turn derives from the nature of things as they are. Perhaps it could have been different, but not in this universe at temperatures and pressures as they presently exist. The universe as we see it is governed by the laws of thermodynamics operating within the physical structure of matter as we understand it. This is the rationalist's intellectual stance: she cannot allow local exceptions. She cannot say: "The laws of thermodynamics are universal except in the cases of wood sprites, oracles and wizards of Class IV and above." So any system we devise to account for our observations of the universe has to be complete in itself. No miracles, without exception, and especially no little miracles to bridge the occasional gap in our thinking. Gaps mean: "Try harder."

Secondly, because the claimed supernatural realm doesn't obey the rules of the natural world, there is no physical means of testing for it just because it doesn't obey the rules of the natural world. While you may believe in ghosts, you will never be able to catch one just because they can slip nimbly through any trap. We cannot devise a meter to measure angelic presences so we can see in the morning if one passed our way during the night. We cannot show that the planets do not exert influences on people at the moment of birth just because our system says that there is no such thing as disembodied information. Information exists as a derivative of the physical world; without its physical substrate, it ceases to exist. No instrument we can invent can be influenced by disembodied information, so we can never have a measure of its effect. In the natural world, there is no true action at a distance and no telepathy. Something else caused it.

The rationalist's starting position is that the world is as it is, and we have to explain the facts as they are. Some people can't accept that, hence we have creation myths. The world consists of matter, energy and information, nothing else. Everything that exists is governed by the laws governing matter, energy and information just because there are no other laws in the natural realm. There is therefore no design: matter, energy and information could not have "designed" themselves because one of them would need to have existed before the others. It could not be information, as there can be no disembodied information but, if the design came first, it would have to exist as information. It could not have designed itself as it requires nothing more than itself to exist. The world is as it is because of the way events have unfolded. For example, if, within a few moments of the Big Bang, the universe hadn't become lumpy, there would be no stars, no planets and therefore none of us. Why are things lumpy? The rationalist looks at clouds and wonders why they clump rather than spreading across the sky as a mist, like air pollution does. If clouds are composed of water vapor, why does it not spread uniformly through the atmosphere? Clouds must have something to do with local temperatures, that's all our rationalist can suggest; but she is sure cloud wraiths have nothing to do with it.

There is no design: nature meanders along its way and we can only explain it after the event. It is feasible that this world could have been devoid of life but each step on the path toward life dramatically increased the odds of the next step happening. Plants greatly increased the levels of oxygen in the atmosphere, thereby increasing the chances of mobile life forms which need a lot of oxygen to move—and which could then move about to use the plants as food. Unlike the Spartoi of Cadmus, nothing springs into life fully formed from nothing. Everything has a prior cause but with a strong random element in it because of the infinite numbers of factors which interact to produce every event. Determinism is impossible because nothing could exist to keep account of and direct the myriad factors that lead me to write this sentence just so and not another way. Given these premises, we are forced to conclude that humans reached their present state without design. It follows that if life can happen on one planet, it can probably happen on others but I don't expect to know the answer in my life time.

If there is no design, nothing can ever deviate from the design. It would follow that, in the materialist world, there can be no notion of paradise, either in the past or the future. The evolutionist says we are not on a road to perfection or away from it, we're not even on a road. We just live in our sandpit with nothing at the beginning and nothing at the end, no Great Sandpit in the Sky. However, the rationalist does not see this as a cause for a Sartrean despair: we are not "forlorn" or "abandoned" in the world, and the lack of an ultimate goal or purpose does not make life "absurd." To the committed materialist, there is no paradise we can earn or attain; if there is no paradise, there is no path to it, or True Path, as people prefer to say. Critically, with no true path (in lowercase), there can be no ordained or universal morality. And if there is no ordained morality, then no person can condemn another based on a Higher Authority; in particular, there can be no priesthood to do the condemning.

Materialism cannot be used to derive universal moral imperatives. It does say that some things are better than others but only in terms of the goals set for them. Goals can always be changed as they didn't come from heaven in a vision (we know that visions are caused by temporal lobe epilepsy). Welcome to life without an angelic long stop. Materialism might have a few bits of its jigsaw still missing, but at least you can see the bigger picture makes sense: "If it made sense, it wouldn't be religion."

This may seem to be a rather roughshod dismissal of some very powerful human institutions but the biocognitive model can give a rational account of many of them. I suggest that religion derives from the innate cognitive system, by means of the sense of awe which derives from contemplating something very powerful. We can get it from watching a huge waterfall, a vast sunrise, a volcano, giant waves or a great animal. We feel it when we see a vast building or some great demonstration of power such as the first nuclear test. When power rests in a man, we feel a sense of awe when nearing him, and not the least because of the danger he represents. If we combine our innate awareness of power with the sense of calm and security that comes from knowing the power will protect us if we follow its rules, we have an explanation for the apparently incessant human drive for something to worship. The term "something to worship" simply means "something vastly powerful that both thrills me and frightens me, something that makes sense of the universe and can protect me." It feels good, it is comforting, so people always seek it. The drive for a "universal comforter" is very deep-seated.

9-2 (b). A theory of humans

Humans are apes and, like our arboreal cousins, we have an innate cognitive system, we do not arrive in the world *tabula rasa*. Instead, we come loaded with preconceptions and prejudices but, because they have always been there and our families seem to share them, we don't see them as prejudices, just normality. Some of our prejudices have a physical basis: we need our daily food and water, we need shelter and something to keep warm; we can't fly or swim very far and we can't walk for hours over hot gravel so we have to stay close to our needs. We don't have strong claws or teeth but our large, color-sensitive eyes with binocular vision mean we can see our enemies before we need to fight them. It all fits in but, if it didn't fit in this way, it would fit in another way.

However, we have better-developed cerebral faculties, such as a capacity to see relationships (and an opposable thumb that allows us to capitalize on them). We learn rapidly and can generalize from single examples. We are socially aggressive and territorial, and we form dominance hierarchies. We have language and a sense of rhythm (we are the only animals that can march in step), meaning we are born with the basic necessities for an army. However, we also have a sense of play and of humor, a sense of curiosity and a fear of strangers and the unknown. We are the only animals that routinely take drugs but we can dream of the ascetic life. We feel a need to explore and explain, we have a sense of fair play but we can be aggressive. Nothing is more exciting than roundly defeating our neighbors, there is no aphrodisiac like victory. In short, we are a mass of contradictions, but each one of them has a role, and its larger purpose was survival in a time when survival wasn't certain. It still isn't. As always, humans are the greatest threat to each other but this time, it is greed, not aggression.

9-2 (c). A universal diagnosis

Materialism denies that there is a universal diagnosis. If we aren't going anywhere, nobody can stray from the path so there can be no universal ailment or malady. There is no Original Sin, no social alienation or anomie and no Great Tempter. This is not a vale of tears because it's the only one we will ever know. There is no paradise (and no hell), no virgins waiting by the cool waters, no endless cycle of birth and rebirth, no universal spirits waiting for us to harmonize with them, no Inner Self yearning to be released and soar into the sunset like Jonathon Livingstone Budgerigar; there is no tarot, no divine light, no prophets, no messiahs, no deliverance, no sacrifices or martyrdom, no UFOs, no alien abduction, no second goes... no magic. This is it.

Does that mean materialism is boring? I don't think so. There is enough in the natural world which is beautiful, fascinating, intriguing, puzzling and inspiring to keep us going for a very long time to come. And for those whose idea of fun doesn't stretch to climbing misty mountains in the pre-dawn darkness to see the sun rise over a rim of volcanoes, there is always music, art, literature, mathematics, cooking, chess and football to while away the hours. But not war, thank you.

9-2 (d). A universal prescription

If there is no ailment, there is no prescription. It would be easy to say, Life is what you make of it but it isn't always true. Christopher Reeve broke his neck, his wife later died of lung cancer. Wealth and connections couldn't help them. Ahmed Mouhrabin's legs were blown off by a suicide bomber as he was coming back from school and he bled to death before his mother found him; a week later, his aunt in Gaza was critically burned by an Israeli phosphorous shell. Twelve year old Charity Murokere was kidnapped by the Lord's Resistance Army and had to provide sex for the troops for fear she would be disemboweled like the other little girl. You know the story.

People at the top of the social pile always attribute their success in life to their superior moral equipment and overlook how lucky they have been. People at the bottom blame the people at the top, especially when they have lost their money drinking or paying for grotesquely expensive weddings. It is women who perform infundibulations on young girls, men who build weapons; women who buy diamond chokers and men who kill for the stones; old people who sell drugs and young people who use them. There is only one universal prescription: we are each responsible for ourselves. Nothing else works. That is the only test because there is no Higher Authority. Well, maybe there is but she's keeping it quiet.

9-3. A Human Reality

Given our physical shape (ape-shape) and our particular sensory organs (rather apish), there isn't much difficulty with the idea that our basic anatomy and physiology was determined by *H. erectus,* and his by *Australopithecus.* Shape is not difficult to explain. More complex matters, such as the results of Harry Harlow's classic experiments with infant rhesus monkeys in the 1950s, will require a different approach. I have outlined a basic model for the innate cognitive system, whereby a sensory input is routed more or less directly to the emotional centers and immediately triggers behavior which is stereotyped just because it is driven by emotion, not by rational needs. The clearest example is very small children laughing at something or being frightened, etc. They don't know what is funny about somebody putting on a silly mask and saying "boo" but it certainly works. With cerebral maturity comes the capacity to over-rule these crude responses but the rapid, intuitive and often socially inappropriate patterns of behavior are never far away. Young boys are quite competitive but the clearest example of pointless competitive behavior is in young adult males, with young adult women a close second. But is it pointless? Or does it confer an advantage in breeding?

For millenia, philosophers have focused their energies on the rational or reasoning side of mental life, largely ignoring the intuitive or unreasoning side. Yet it is the latter which causes us so much trouble such as fighting, the vast expenditure of resources on matters of pride, the endless quest for emotional security in ceremony and ritual, etc. If we wish to secure our future, we need to take it much more seriously.

Consider a small example of a major problem. Once aroused, humans have no means of turning off aggression except defeat. Strictly hierarchical social animals such as wolves and baboons can defuse aggression by adopting a submissive posture whereas for territorial animals, the aggressive drive normally switches off only when the angry animal crosses the borders of its territory. This can be seen in doves or quail, which are highly territorial but have no social structure as such. If a pair of quail are released in a suitable cage and allowed to establish themselves, then introducing another quail will result in the resident pair attacking it. In the bush, the newcomer would simply skip to safety across the border of the resident pair's territory. However, in the cage, the newcomer has no means of escape. The resident birds will attack it, and keep on attacking it, until it dies, just because they have no other behavioral response to an intruder. Humans are also highly territorial and have no innate capacity to switch off aggression. As traditional Australian Aboriginal society showed [2], a stranger would be attacked unless and until he fled across the border to his own tribe's territory. There was nothing he could do to stop this, not gifts, pleas or submission. As an intruder, there was only one choice awaiting him: run, or die.

So, when humans are crammed together with no means of escape, the weakest have no way of deflecting aggression. This is highly significant in urban life, which was not the social structure that obtained during our evolution (essentially, all modern life is urban). It means that, where there are disputed borders, tribal warfare will continue to rage because the normal mechanism of defusing the aggressive impulse, crossing into a stranger's territory, is no longer operative. The victors in wars will storm across the vanquished tribe's territory in an orgy of blood and sex, experiencing no diminution of their aggression akin to that felt by the defeated warriors. It is for this reason that humans *en masse* have turned into mass murderers. We have no innate mechanism for stopping the slaughter of the innocents. There is clear archeological evidence that this has always been the case [3].

9-4. A Humanist Morality

If there is no Higher Authority available to us, then where does that leave morality? What is morality? *Morality:* Noun, 1. the quality of being moral; 2. a system of morals; 3. conforming to conventional standards of moral conduct... *Moral:* adj. 1. concerning or relating to human behavior, esp. the distinction between good and bad or right and wrong behavior...

The question becomes this: in the absence of a Higher Authority, can there ever be a rational system of moral behavior? Are there universal standards of morality or is all behavior relative? These are ancient questions but, fortunately, they are not my field. My concern is only with the natural humanist model derived in the earlier chapters as I have a proprietary interest to ensure that nobody ever tries to use this model to impose their views on other people. That is not its purpose.

Can this model of human nature generate a general set of morals? The first point is that, if it did, the system would be as close to universal as we have ever seen, just because it derives from the common features of humans, not unique features of one particular culture. Are there already universal elements of morality genetically encoded in every human that ever existed? I don't believe I have ever seen an example of a supposedly universal moral imperative which was not, somewhere, at some time, contradicted by some other culture [4]. If morality is divorced from a particular cosmic view, there can be no such thing as a chosen race or a priestly caste. There can be no wars based on "We are morally superior to you and we're going to kill you to prove it." Morals might, of course, vary for local reasons but everybody would know that these are simply matters of local convenience and not to be imposed at gunpoint upon the people from the next valley. This might not be seen as an improvement by those who habitually expect others to share their views.

The second point to ponder is what purpose morality serves. If is just to entrench the power of the priests or the army, then we would be better off without it. However, I don't believe that is the case. The role of a moral system is to regulate behavior, to prevent anarchy on a small or large scale. Ideally, we therefore need only choose our goals and a system of morality will declare itself. So what is the goal in a humanist, materialist system? Make sure you survive. If you have an eye for the future, you might like to add: "...long enough to breed." However, a solipsistic system is unstable; *Macht hat Recht* is fine until somebody comes along with more Macht than your Recht. So we trade off certain options in return for some sort of stability. We need to recall that, in all practicality, we have to assume that this is the only world with life, so we need to be rather careful what we do with it. It is reported that, during the countdown to the Trinity blast on July 16th 1945, Enrico Fermi wondered whether the impending explosion would ignite the atmosphere. Was that the first real awareness that we have the power to destroy the only life we know? Nowadays, anybody who can read is aware that we are risk of causing irremediable damage to the biosphere, whereas that thought may not have occurred to another soul during the whole of World War II. So perhaps this is the ultimate purpose of any moral system: that we have a duty to preserve this unique experiment called life. What consequences flow from this position?

Without arguing the case, because it drifts too far from my purpose, a very great deal flows from it. We have a duty to live in such a manner as to ensure, for example, that we will still be here, in much the same world in, say, three hundred years. That's much less than the time since white settlement in North America, only eighty years longer than the first European colony in Australia. It isn't long but if we are pumping three million tons of carbon dioxide into the atmosphere every hour, and the consumption of fossil fuels is likely to double in less than thirty years, will we make it to 2309? Purely coincidentally, the European winter of 1709-10, i.e. just 300 years ago, was the worst for many hundreds of years. Directly and indirectly, it caused the deaths of over a million people. That says we can't argue with Mother Nature.

Without examining the question closely, I incline to the view that a fully sustainable lifestyle is inconsistent with the doctrine of Winner takes All. I see greed as destabilizing and excessively risky, leading to arms races and the destruction of resources by military activity. Many other activities would fail the test of sustainability, such as extravagant weddings and funerals, commercial sport and other forms of inequitable consumption. But is economic durability the only goal? A lot of other habits, such as circumcision and subincision, enforced marriages or denial of contraception, flow from a perverse social structure where power derives from a particular ontology and is distributed unequally through the society. A great deal of dispute and disharmony derives from the flashpoints along the borders of different power structures; these lead to posturing (same as chimps) and all too often to arms races and fighting (chimps with nuclear weapons), with all that that entails. So in order to ensure sustainability, we may need to revise inequitable social systems, except that will still not stop posturing and threat displays, because they may well be innate. However, we don't need to stop them, just control them. We can't stop flatus, but there's no need to worship it.

Yet behind any contractual agreement to lead a sustainable lifestyle lies the threat of force to prevent backsliding; that is inescapable. There is very little cause for optimism that the whole of the human race will agree on a single course of action just because it seems sensible. As long as there are humans with opinions, there will be differences of opinion. The totalitarian response, to eradicate all opinions except one, is unstable; better we should learn how to reconcile differences, trading them away while still keeping an eye on the longer-term goal. But in order to do that successfully, we need a formal model of mind which takes rational account of the irrationalities of human nature, or the innate cognitive system, which is where this model may be of use.

It should be understood that sustainability does not flow from the model itself. It derives from a value we place on the continuation of what seems a very, very rare experiment in life, maybe even unique. There is no moral value inherent in the biocognitive model itself; it isn't that sort of thing. Just as the periodic table or the genome of *E. coli* are devoid of values, so too is the biocognitive model. It is a theoretical model to explain how things are but it does not say: This is how things *ought* to be. Value is a human construct; this model tries to explain that construct—without placing any value on it.

9-5. A Theory Of Society

It will be clear that certain elements in this model do have sociological implications. Where empirical facts conflict with normative systems, humans will suffer or the system will have to change. For example, in Australia's Northern Territory, the Aboriginal community is urged to live as close to their traditional lifestyle as they like. However, this immediately causes conflict with the Western system as many elements of traditional Aboriginal society breach major international treaties which this country has signed. For example, traditional society is totemic, which determines who the individual must marry. Women are chattels who belong to their appointed husbands. If an old man's wife dies, he can take a young bride, even if she is barely pubertal and occasionally younger [1]. This causes disputes because, in the Western view, this amounts to rape of a child, a very serious offence as minors are deemed incapable of consenting. Should the old man go to prison or should he not? They are, as lawyers complain on behalf of the girls. Similarly, if the girl runs off with a young man, the old man can compel him to undergo ritual spearing, consisting of shoving up to half a dozen (dirty) wooden spears in through one of the younger man's legs and out through the other. He is left skewered for an hour or two, and then they are removed.

Even if the young man consents to his ritual punishment, should the old man be sent to prison for doing what his culture ordains? They never are, as the young men dare not complain.

Similarly, there is enormous pressure on adolescent boys to undergo tribal circumcision, a singularly unpleasant procedure performed by short-sighted old men using a sharp rock or a sharp shell in their tremulous and anything but sanitary hands. The wounded organ is wrapped in fresh mud to aid the healing process. If the youth refuses, he is not classed as a man and therefore cannot have a wife. In some areas, he is further expected to undergo subincision, in which the penile urethra is laid open for a length of about four or five centimeters, again with a sharp shell. This grotesque procedure is not compulsory but the pressure to conform is such that very few young men can resist. All of this flows from a particular religious view of the universe which, as with all other religious ontologies, has no empirical support whatsoever. So is there a place for a culture that generates intolerable pressures that were only constrained by ferocious enforcement of the death penalty? [2]. These are not trivial questions. I suggest answers can be derived from a model of society as a collection of individuals needing to reconcile diverse needs, some genetic and some rational, rather than as a reflection of, say, God's immutable will (as received by a small group of old men).

For the record, traditional Aboriginal culture had many institutions which other cultures regard as abhorrent. There were trials by sorcery, secret trials for capital charges which the accused never knew about until his executioners struck, infanticide and gerontocide, terrible corporal punishment, ritual mutilation, and sexual abasement of women including ritual cleansing after childbirth so they could again provide sexual relations for their appointed husbands. There was no choice in any of this. Breaches of traditional law carried immediate, brutal punishments with no right of appeal, etc. None of this is compatible with even the most basic of agreed human rights. Also for the record, traditional Western society hasn't been any better throughout most of its recorded history. Whether it is now remains open to debate.

This raises the crucial point: to what extent can a society be permitted to govern the lives of its citizens, including non-citizens such as children, prisoners and mental patients. Should Arab women wear purdah and accept second-rate status in courts? Should the Taliban blow up irreplaceable ancient Buddhist statues? Should Western bankers take home hundreds of millions of dollars a year while taxpayers prop up their bankrupt businesses? Should the Grand Bank cod fishery be fished to desolation, Iran build a nuclear power station for "energy security" while daily flaring vast quantities of natural gas? Should the Chinese be in Tibet, the Indonesians in West Papua, the Americans everywhere? These are not trivial questions but they go to the heart of the notion of a sustainable, civil society. I do not want my children to face life in a mortally wounded planet, a matter over which they had no control but for which they will carry full responsibility long after today's billionaires and politicians are dead.

A naturalist model of mind generates answers to these questions, some of them direct, more of them indirect. Does this matter? It does. Religion has signally failed to promote fair and equitable societies, historicist doctrines like communism and fascism were among the world's worst, nationalism is a cancer which eats men's vitals, racism and tribalism fuel the very worst excesses, oligarchy simply delays the day of reckoning, and so on. There is no question whatsoever that humans are social animals with strong hierarchical and territorial urges. If we combine the social urge with territoriality, the direct outcome is the tribe, or nation-state when it gets big enough. That wouldn't matter if we were not also xenophobic, but this extra factor will inevitably lead to friction where one tribe abuts another. The problem is that humans really can be grotesquely awful when the mood strikes them, and they are at their worst when they think they are right. But that is a truism: we always think we are right. We cannot believe something we know to be wrong, therefore, whatever we do we justify. This is a product of our nature as higher primates. For a civil society, the issue is not to pretend that this won't happen, although one would have thought history should have provided a hint, but to institute suitable safety mechanisms that will channel and defuse the tension before the bombs start flying.

Similarly, we can talk about the equality of the sexes but if it were a fact, then we wouldn't need legislation to guarantee it. The sexes are not equal, the physiological and psychological evidence is overwhelming; we need to take these differences into account, and not set up irreconcilable tensions within young people to conform to what is little more than ideological fantasy. Widespread and historical pressures for people to conform to social mores, such as the ancient prohibitions on homosexuality, should be examined in a humanist context and not measured against the traditions of, say, Leviticus. Indeed, a "work-to-rule" based on the Old Testament would be farcical. For example, it is not widely known that it sanctions incest, but only in cases where the tribe is likely to die out (see what happened to Lot the night after Sodom was destroyed, Gen. 19: 30-38).

We can discuss these issues at great length, but it would help if we could come to some decision before the polar icecaps melt.

9-6. A Theory of Law

The idea of a law-governed society tends not to attract those of us brought up in the permissive sixties and seventies. Indeed, such a society is often vilified as wantonly destructive and anti-humanitarian, a callous and brutal means of separating people from their inner spiritual selves and turning them into robotic slaves of the consumerist society. Or something. On the other hand, the basis of a civil human society must be start with the nature of the beast, and the nature of the beast is, well, pretty beastly. Short of utopia, a rule-governed society may be the only way that rule-driven creatures can ever hope to live together in passable harmony and fulfillment. We are creatures of habit: while anarchy may give a few young men the chance to indulge their need for physical dominance, it scares most people, especially children.

The question to be answered here is how to find a reasonable balance between individual freedoms and group security. My concern is not the actual laws that people implement, or system of laws, but the fundamental notions that inform such systems. For example, it may be that, after the dispassionate application of a number of principles deriving from the nature of the planet and the nature of humans, some societies conclude that the only rational response to certain crimes is the death penalty. The point is to separate law from morality. Capital punishment after due process might be abhorrent to some but it would be an advance on systems of laws that demand death by stoning for women who have been raped. Civil law must never derive from a prior morality; that puts the cart before the horse. Furthermore, using carefully determined empirical principles as the basis for a legal system would go a long way to prevent government by pressure groups. For example, the double standard of legalizing alcohol while banning marihuana has no rational or practical basis whatsoever. Sir Percival Pott said: "If there is one thing which infallibly distinguishes man from the other animals, it is the enduring proclivity of the former to consume all manner of drugs."

The tendency of humans to use psychoactive drugs is a product of our psychophysiology. Whether it is desirable or not, it is not going to stop by legislation. Therefore, control by regulation, rather than futile attempts to dictate to people who have no intention of being dictated to, is the only rational response. The folly of prohibition is best seen in comparing different cultures. For example, most Western governments ban marihuana and expect their citizens to follow the rules dutifully. At the same time, they are eagerly encouraging citizens living under some very nasty regimes to oppose their governments in word and deed. This duplicity seems a little unrealistic and self-serving, at least. Other quintessentially human activities, such as fighting, prostitution and gambling, will also not be controlled by legislation, just because they are such fun, and fun is crudely biological, not coolly rational. Sean Flynn said we will never stop war as it is too sexy (that was before he was captured by the Khmer Rouge and tortured to death). Combining our drive for dominance with the excitement generated by fighting produces an unstable cocktail of unthinking impulses. For young men, winning is the most powerful aphrodisiac of all. For young women, there is nothing so sexually arousing as a triumphant young man: he just smells so good. A major focus of every legal/moral system since the beginning of recorded time has been controlling base human passions, but these equate with the primitive urges we inherited as part of our primate nature. These urges don't listen to reason, just because they aren't plugged into the same system.

Gambling is a potent attraction for humans, both men and women. The current financial collapse has arisen because people gambled against the possibility of economic disaster—and lost, just because their gambling created the disaster they believed couldn't happen. Unfortunately, this was after they had managed to draw into their high-stakes game many hundreds of millions of ordinary people who were never asked whether they wanted anyone to gamble with their limited assets. We will simply not stop people gambling on the stock exchange (or horses, or cards), the excitement is overwhelming, but, as fast as governments try to limit it, the gamblers will find ways of slipping through. Gambling is about winning, and the excitement of winning is programmed into us by millions of years of evolution. Devising a financial system which separated the gamblers from cautious, long-term investors would not be difficult and would go a long way to preventing repetitions of our present woes. Unfortunately, it would be bitterly opposed by the bankers and financiers as "unworkable," not because it is unworkable but just because it would spoil their fun. The whole point of playing the stock market is to have lots of other people who aren't quite so clever or informed or cutthroat who hand over their money for the clever people to play with. Without trillions of dollars from Mom and Pop investors to manipulate, hedge funds and all the other gimmicks just don't work. Bernard Madoff didn't bilk clever investors, just the slow and greedy. These are the sorts of questions that a formal model of mind can and must address.

9-7. Conclusion

A rational system of laws must take into account the nature of the creatures it is hoping to contain, and the goals it is hoping to achieve within the limits of that nature. There is a human nature, and it isn't very nice. History's endlessly futile attempts to base legal systems on unjustifiable moral imperatives from a fantastic past suggests we could do worse than look to a system based on a rational theory of the human mind. In this respect, the value of the biocognitive model lies in the basic premises it generates. From these flows a system of rules which have a larger purpose than simply maintaining inequitable power structures.

Part III: Applying the Biocognitive Model to Psychiatry

10 The Role of Personality

"This impression of scientific certitude in the midst of substantial and potentially crippling problems is a tribute to the ability of psychologists and the psychiatric profession to acquire and wield power."
Eric T Dean

10-1. Introduction

In psychiatry, personality is all. This immediately puts me at odds with orthodox psychiatry but I will not apologize: biological psychiatry doesn't even have a model of personality. That is not from a shortage of models but from intellectual sloth. Modern psychiatrists believe they have mental disorder in an arm lock, that it is only a matter of time before molecular biochemistry churns out the answers to the few remaining bits and pieces so we can dive into a brave new world of tailor-made drugs—for all people, for all reasons and seasons (but will politicians take their tablets, too?).

Personality disorder is one of those irksome bits and pieces, but one which doesn't interest orthodox psychiatrists. Indeed, a convincing case could be made for a powerful sociological trend in which psychiatrists are no longer diagnosing personality disorder. Instead, the mournful, the misfits and the obstreperous get shiny diagnostic labels such as ADD/ADHD, Bipolar Affective Disorder Type II or (better still) Comorbid Dysthymic Disorder and Social Phobia with Substance Abuse. This trend opens the door to untold millions of people around the world being prescribed long-term drugs for conditions which, traditionally, psychiatrists knew weren't going to get better anyway. They can also go to hospital or to various programs where they learn relaxation or anger management, self-centering or sexual hygiene. This provides employment for very large numbers of psychologists, social workers, therapists, nurses, counselors, administrators, cleaners, accountants and, of course, lawyers. The results are poor but this leads to the usual cries of "more of the same" (more money and jobs) which politicians cannot resist.

The corporatization of medicine proceeds apace, driven by imperatives which are nowhere based in a formal theory of mental disorder. These days, there is no financial incentive to diagnose a personality disorder as the insurers know these people do not change so their treatment is rationed. Diagnoses of formal mental illness, on the other hand, are subsidized, meaning psychiatrists are under intense pressure from the hospitals and from the patients and their families to find a diagnosis no matter what the cost. This is also true of the compensation industry, where today's disturbance is laid at the feet of some obscure incident many years before: *post hoc, ergo propter hoc*, so pay up.

That, however, is modern psychiatry. Antediluvian psychiatry—the sort I studied so many years ago—was in no stronger position, not because we had no models of personality but because we had too many. We didn't have anything like a course in personality theory or, as people now say, a metatheory of personality. Instead, trainees were "exposed" to the competing models in a random process spread over the course of several years. This meant we picked up snippets of these totally incompatible notions buried in courses on other topics. So, we heard about the Freudian model of personality during a brief and chaotic series of lectures on psychoanalytic theory by an odd lady who, we agreed, might once have read Calvin Hall's *Primer of Freudian Psychology*. The behaviorist concept of personality was given as an afterthought by a psychologist who clearly saw teaching trainee psychiatrists as supping with the devil. Our "exposure" to the biological concept of personality was given *en passant* by a committed biological psychiatrist who regarded personality disorder as a moral failing, while I nodded off during the lecture on cognitive psychology and must have missed personality.

In those days, I was still inclined to believe that our lecturers actually knew what they were talking about. That meant I was left juggling four or more utterly contradictory approaches to an undefined field that the lecturers had dismissed in a few words. Now, of course, I know better: personality is of profound importance, and psychiatrists (and psychologists, and all the rest) know nothing about it. Nothing.

10-2. Models of Personality?

10-2 (a). Failed models of personality

We can dispense with three of the four classes of personality theories fairly quickly. Reductionist biological psychiatry has nothing to say about normal personality. Biological psychiatrists approach the intuitive concept of personality disorder from the same categorical viewpoint that drives their appraisal of all mental disorder, by sorting it into clusters as a prelude to assigning separate biochemical lesions to each cluster. This, of course, is mere promissory materialism of a fairly low order. As I have shown, not only are the DSM-IV groups of personality disorder feeble and unable to counter the slightest criticism but they also stand in an intellectual vacuum. Reductive biologism does not have a rational concept of personality which would, in turn, generate the classes of personality disorder. Notions of dependent or aggressive personalities float free in an undefined conceptual space. This means, of course, that everybody can happily get on with the business of prescribing drugs (or breathing techniques, or rebirthing) completely unencumbered by moral notions of whether we ought to be doing this. My view is that, by ignoring personality, by translating it into illness, orthodox psychiatry is creating enormous problems for its patients—and for itself.

My first exposure to Freudian theories of personality was very early in my training. In those days, there was only one book on Freudian theory to read, Otto Fenichel's *The Psychoanalytic Theory of Neurosis*. Also in those days, in the world's most isolated capital city, there was just copy available to trainees, so we could only borrow it for a month. As a late starter in the program, I was at the end of the queue. As my intention in psychiatry was to become a psychoanalyst, I eagerly awaited my turn. Almost every other day, I heard amazed comments from the others in my group as they ploughed through it. Finally, I was next. Week after week, I listened to my lucky colleague as he recounted to me what a brilliant work of science it was, how its astounding insights opened an entirely new perspective on the human condition. He kept it an extra week, I recall, then I had it in my hands and could finally set to work on my career. However, after only a few pages, I had serious doubts about the whole deal. It seemed to me that nobody had the right to make the unjustified claims that stuffed each turgid page. I read to page 29 then I took it back, greatly troubled by my inescapable feeling that it was just high-sounding nonsense. Everything I have learned since then reinforces my early, inchoate objections.

In those days, of course, I could not put my intuitions into words as I didn't have the education. We were not trained in critical thinking, and medical education was certainly not based in the idea that the greats needed criticizing, especially by students. Thus, when an influential author says: "...psychoanalysis still represents the most coherent and intellectually satisfying view of the mind" [1, p64], it is clear that one of us (or both) is wrong. In fact, as we now know, it is the psychoanalytic apologist who, wholly for the wrong reasons, has been blinded by his "first love" [2]. Not only is psychoanalytic theory non-scientific, it is incapable of being transformed into an empirical field. With all due respect to elderly neurophysiologists, time has consigned Freud's masterpiece to the history books.

Since the rest of this chapter is about a cognitive theory of personality, I don't need to say more just now. First, I will look at some of the problems of the behaviorist approach to personality because they bear directly on modern psychiatric practice.

10-2 (b). What is a behaviorist model of personality?

Almost at the end of his career, H.J. Eysenck, one of the most influential of twentieth century behaviorists who had devoted a very large part of his remarkably productive life to the theory of personality, was moved to admit he had not achieved his life's goal of writing a theory of personality. He did not even have a model of personality, just an idea of what a model of personality might be like. For Eysenck, personality could not include any mention of irrefutable inner states, such as mind. Thus, in the behaviorist schema, personality is simply a constellation of dispositions to act in certain ways. The individual's dispositions are determined by asking him questions about how he habitually acts and feels. Because behaviorists wanted their work to be immune to the vagaries of the interviewer's own dispositions, they used standardized questions which statistical analysis had shown would yield the maximum information.

There are different ways this can be done. One of the most influential questionnaires was assembled over many years by Raymond Cattell, who used the Allport-Odbert lists of some 18,000 personality terms derived from dictionaries of the English language. Cattell then submitted these lists to factor analysis and derived sixteen primary factors which further clustered into five groups, the so-called "Big Five Factors." Cattell's 16PF, as it is generally known, grades individuals on each of his primary factors, giving a global assessment of personality style. For example, a person who scores highly on Warmth is socially-involved, concerned, outgoing and generally likes to be with people. A low-scorer is reserved, socially-distant, detached, cool and uninvolved. A person who scores low in Dominance is submissive, humble, easily led, docile and accommodating, while a high-scorer is dominant, competitive to the point of aggression, forceful and assertive and often stubborn.

The Big Five or global factors vary somewhat from one research group to another, but there is general agreement that they involve Openness, Conscientiousness, Extraversion, Agreeableness and Neuroticism, usually abbreviated to OCEAN. These are clusters of behaviors, in which the elements of each cluster are more like each other than they are like members of any other cluster. Each major factor is composed of a number of lesser-order factors. A person who scores high in one subscore of a major factor is likely to score highly on the others, and so on. Eysenck was convinced there were only three major factors but he seems to have lost that round.

Behaviorist theories of personality lead inexorably to one question: So what? How does it help us to know that a person is high on Agreeableness if all we have done is ask him? How does it advance our knowledge of him? This is the major objection to behaviorist approaches to personality, that they say nothing about the unseen mechanisms which generate observable behavior, meaning they are not theories of personality but typologies of personality. Thus, the questionnaires may indicate that Mr. A is socially distant and avoidant without revealing that he is highly anxious and has terrible self-esteem. Ms. B, on the other hand, is socially distant and avoidant because she firmly believes she is better than most people and, if she lets them get too close, they will prevent her pursuing her goals and standards. Granted this is a crude example but it shows that visible behavior can have many different causes: the causes are forever hidden to a behaviorist.

Furthermore, what benefit comes from knowing this is how a person is likely to act in different situations? In psychiatry, we are really concerned with changing behavior. So the behaviorist model is of no benefit unless it can be tied to some underlying mechanism which is then amenable to intervention. Traditionally, behaviorists hoped their typologies could be tied to genetics, that personality was essentially a matter of inheritance but this has not been a productive line of research. If there are genetic contributions to personality, they are exceedingly complex and highly interactive with the environment. In addition, genes code for proteins, and no reasonable person would claim we yet have a model of how proteins cause people to be "sensitive, esthetic, sentimental, tender-minded, intuitive, refined" (high Sensitivity) or "tolerant of disorder, unexacting, flexible, undisciplined, careless of social rules, impulsive, uncontrolled and lacking self-conflict" (low Perfectionism). There has to be a hidden mechanism to bridge the gap, something that reaches from proteins to estheticism and, critically, vice versa. A theory defines a potential path where none is obvious.

Despite its preoccupation with being good science, behaviorist typologies of personality have not been able to relate behavior to anything internal. Partly this is because they eschewed mentalism and partly because they have no solution to the mind-body problem (or brain-behavior problem, as they prefer to say). That is, they left themselves no bridge between genes and behavior. Perhaps this is why psychologists are quietly drifting away from the idea that defined them for a hundred years. Why were they convinced in the first place? "A clear utopian message, hammered home relentlessly, will obscure inconvenient facts" [3].

10-3. The Biocognitive Model of Personality

10-3 (a). A theory of personality

A theory is a suggestion of an unseen mechanism which could generate the observations in question. This is an example of a theory:

- Observed fact 1: Gold is found in the earth's crust.

- Observed fact 2: Gold can only be formed under conditions of great temperature and pressure.

- Observed fact 3: Suitable conditions of temperature and pressure are only found in stars.

- Theory: All the gold on earth arose in a star, but not our sun or any complete star as it could not have escaped the stellar gravitational field. Therefore it must have come from the wreckage of another star.

A theory is not a fact. A theory is a cluster of suggestions embedded in a larger belief system which amount to a possible mechanism that could explain the observations.

Here is another example of a theory:

- Observed fact 1: Human behavior is goal-directed.

- Observed fact 2: Molecules do not have goals.

- Theory: Something other than molecules causes human behavior.

In the case of humans, the biocognitive model states that the "something other" that causes observable behavior consists of rules coded at the level of the molecular function of specific CNS neurons. The information contained in the rules is able to act directly upon the efferent neurons of the motor and secretomotor nuclei of the CNS, such that detailed instructions are sent to the effector organs resulting in coherent, goal-directed behavior. While it would be very helpful if we could be sure of the brain's codes, this is not necessary as we can use a shorthand to characterize them, just as we do with any modern machine with data processing capabilities.

For example, I can say of my car: "It will tell me if a door isn't closed properly."

This does not mean that the vehicle "knows" (in any interesting sense of the word) when a door is unlatched, but it does mean there is a dumb mechanism built into the frame whose net effect is to light a lamp on the dash when a door is unlatched. The car doesn't "tell" me anything, it doesn't even "know" when there is a person inside it, or what a door is. Cars aren't bright enough to tell humans from bananas, meaning they don't have the specific detectors nor do they have enough computing power to compute a valid decision from those detectors.

So if I want to explain to you just what I mean by "The car will tell me if a door isn't closed properly," I have to start with the idea of a circuit built into the door frame which lights a lamp on the dash board if and only if the circuit is not closed. That is, I must invoke the concept of a logic gate, specifically the unary operator or "not" gate described in Chap. 6. I could say to you: "There is a special circuit built into each door and wired to the dash such that a light will show on the dash if and only if the door is not locked properly. The wiring consists of 100mg copper minicircuits connected to a Smithson VLX AB66F microprocessor, where lead A is connected to the driver's door and lead B... etc." Since that's a bit of a mouthful, I lazily say: "It will tell me if a door isn't closed properly." When you hear that, you do not conclude that modern cars come equipped with brains and souls because you just know that I am ducking the technical stuff. In the interests of brevity, we agree to attribute to the car the same mental attributes we would attribute to a person who performed the same function: he would tell me: "Hey, your door's open." Even if the car had a speaker that yelled out "Hey, stupid, your door's open," it wouldn't be telling me that as it can only "tell" me. That sentence summarizes how the intact machine takes in the information and what it does with it. As long as we never forget that we have to give an elemental account of how that information is gathered, processed and effected, we are legitimately able to use the shorthand. The same goes for the information coded into the human brain. Because we don't know where it is coded or the codes themselves, we simply use a shorthand which, one day, might be rendered in explicit, electromechanical form but, then again, might not be. Whether it ever is or isn't does not bother us because psychiatrists aren't so much interested in the minutiae of the specific codes but the impact of the information they carry. So, if you are scared of frogs, I don't need to know the precise instantaneous state of every neuron involved in you feeling a sudden jolt of fear, all I have to do is say, "I see you're scared of frogs." That sentence summarizes how the intact human takes in the information and what he does with it. As long as we never forget that, one day, we will have to give a sub-neuronal account of how that information is gathered, processed and effected, we are legitimately able to use the shorthand. At this point, you might raise an objection: Isn't this just biological reductionism recast in modern jargon? No, not at all, because reductionism denies the causative efficacy of the non-physical realm of data-processing. I am saying that information processing is the causally efficacious realm in human behavior, which is precisely the opposite of what biological psychiatry claims is the case.

By this means, I believe it is legitimate to characterize the individual's coded rules in his native language, even though we know the brain does not operate in native languages. It operates in brain languages, and then in virtual machine languages, but we can recast them in, say, English just so long as we are fully aware that we are concealing stupendous complexity under a simple expression such as: "I see you're scared of frogs." When we get to something like: "Yes, he's a real perfectionist," the complexity of the coded rules that generate that particular behavioral repertoire would overwhelm any modern serial supercomputer. But that's the advantage of having a multi-channel, distributed parallel data processor filling the rather small space between my ears: it can compute very clever answers in milliseconds, and all without causing my feet to stumble.

10-3 (b). A theory of personality as rules

In the biocognitive model, the theory of personality is just this: the entire constellation of coded rules which act to generate observable behavior. Chap. 13 of *Psychiatry and the cognitive neurosciences,* shows how personality should be seen as the sum total of distinguishing rules governing our behavior. Using the "shorthand" described above, these rules can be characterized as simple injunctions in the individual's native tongue: Always repay debts; Never trust strangers; A place for everything and everything in its place; Anything I can do isn't worth much; and so on. Roughly speaking, these rules form two groups, those relating to how the individual sees the world and how he believes it should run, and those relating to how he sees himself as a person and what he should do. We say a person has a normal personality when his set of rules is internally consistent and meshes smoothly with the world and the people around him. If, however, his set of rules is internally inconsistent, causing him fluctuating distress and bringing him into conflict with the natural and human environment, then we say he has a personality disorder. A question immediately arises: how can we relate the concept of personality as a set of rules driving behavior to the empirical evidence of traits such as the Big Five or Cattell's sixteen factors? The answer is: with no difficulty.

We acquire our notion of regularities in the world very early, with such ease that we can characterize humans as creatures that extract rules or suck generalizations from the social and natural worlds. We start this process at a very young age. Bearing in mind that infants go through typical phases of reacting to the world, they are nonetheless starting to show characteristic patterns of behavior by the time they take their first steps. Some of these may well be part of the innate cognitive system, and some hereditary dispositions to particular emotional responses. For example, very early in life, infants of many species demonstrate differential levels of field dependence vs. field independence. The field independent infant explores boldly, even moving right out of sight of its mother, whereas the dependent infant clings anxiously to familiarity. Anxiety is the intervening variable; high anxiety inhibits exploration while low anxiety leads the child into danger. Early interactions between the child and the environment are colored by inherent dispositions to anxiety, and these shape personality for all time. Good parenting in secure surroundings may well be able to overcome the genetic tendency to high anxiety (field dependence), while a child with low inherited anxiety or high independence may swing to the other extreme because of unfavorable early life experiences. Later life experiences may further complicate the early tendencies. This type of interaction is probably sufficient in itself to confound a lot of the early research on genetically-inherited traits of, for example, the British school of behaviorism that formed around Eysenck.

As the child matures, it gains more and more rules from the differing experiences coming its way. These are shaped by the environment and, in turn, shape the environment itself. Bad experiences compound themselves but good times are easily overwhelmed. We are biased toward acquiring rules that guarantee survival, even at the expense of common sense or consistency. Fear is the most powerful teacher of all: one fright can undo half a lifetime of warm experiences because a person in a state of heightened arousal learns more acutely than somebody in a relaxed state. Parenting is of major significance, as all children go through anxious phases. It is the parents' job to guide the child through these phases but anxious parents are not good at this task. They tend to see ordinary life settings as frightening and do not question the child's anxious responses. They may in fact justify it so that the child never learns not to expect danger. Given the inherent tendency to anxiety, it is clear that early life experiences can make the child better or worse than the parental genetic endowment would indicate.

Manifestly, the generalizations relating to the world and their role in it which children acquire from their experience are infinite. Every child is born into a family but the physical circumstances vary enormously, from Windsor Palace to the gutters of Mogadishu. The child's health may be enviable or heart-rending. Intelligence ranges from genius to barely functional. The parental figures, if there are any, may range from caring and considerate to infanticidal brutes. Education may be individualized in a highly supportive school, or a grim matter of survival of the fittest on the streets of Bombay. Finally, life experiences may be gilded or shattered by war or famine. Out of this cocktail comes the functioning or dysfunctional adult. There is no limit to the permutations and combinations of rules with which an individual reaches adulthood.

Even the old saw, that children from the same family have the same developmental experiences, breaks down under the briefest examination. Consider the following case, absolutely typical of a week's work. The subject is a 52yo professional man who has recently experienced a mild stroke and has been unable to work:

> "People don't understand what my life was like. They say, 'Oh, you've got two degrees, a lovely wife, you're lucky,' but I worked my arse off for everything I've got.' I was the second of four children in a country town, all born within six years of each other. For whatever reason, my father favored my older brother, who could do no wrong. In those days, kids were belted if they did anything wrong. My father freely boasted that he had hit me ten times as much as the others put together but it was more like a hundred times. My older brother got three beltings in his life, I know that. My sister got one slap from my mother when she stole something and my little brother was never once

hit. I used to get a flogging every week but I never really knew why. If I'd ever hit my children the way I was hit, I would've gone to prison, and rightly so. I was belted with whatever came to hand. A length of black rubber hose hung behind the door and he would grab me and drag me to the laundry and thrash me until he couldn't hit any more. Another favorite was a stirrup leather from one of his old work saddles, or a jockey whip. He used an electric cord for some time but the welts took days to fade and it was embarrassing for them at church so he gave up on it. Another winner was the rubber ring out of an old pressure cooker, my god, that hurt. You didn't go back for a second round of that.

"But my father also made fun of me, he taunted me and mocked me, and he was at his worst in front of visitors. Maybe I wasn't the best behaved kid in town but I sure wasn't the worst. My marks at school were always top of my year, without fail. My older brother clearly had brains but his results were woeful, he never lifted a finger at school, always had a lie to tell why he hadn't finished his homework. My father told me a dozen times I wasn't as smart as my brother, he would go far but I'd have to settle for a job in a bank. I never got the cane at school, I was never suspended, I was chosen to give speeches to visitors or recite poems but I was no good at sport. My brother was strong and stocky but I was very small and skinny. Of the four children, my marks in the matriculation (university entrance exams) were five times higher than the rest of them put together. My older brother failed outright twice but my marks were the best ever recorded in that town and have never been beaten in that school's eighty years of records. Did I get anything for that? Nothing. My brother had a room full of trophies for sport but I never got so much as a bookmark for my academic results. I have hated flash sportsmen to this day.

"If that wasn't enough, my older brother used to bash the crapper out of me whenever he got the chance. He would knuckle me hard as I walked past but if I yelled out, my old man would wallop me, then my brother would get me again later that day. He would belt me over nothing, really nasty, torturous beltings, he hid my things and taunted and teased me until I went mad but I couldn't tell my parents or I'd get two more floggings, one from my father and another from him. We were in the same school for over half my time at school but he would never talk to me, he never so much as looked at me. He certainly never helped me in any way or stuck up for me if I got into a fight, not that I did very much. He went one way to school, to meet his mates so they could smoke before school, and he made me go another way. We don't look alike, I take after my mother's family and he takes after my father's, and nobody knew we were brothers. People thought we might have been cousins but that's all. No, that wasn't all. My brother used me for sex, two or three times a week for six or seven years. There was no violence because I knew better than to argue. I lived in mortal dread that my father would find out because I knew he would kill me. I mean, kill me. Shoot me like he had shot an injured dog. My brother didn't have anybody to punch his head in a couple of times a week but that is how I grew up. We had separate lives and we've gone separate ways."

10-3 (c). Rules conscious and not-so-conscious

Out of this, the child arrives at adulthood equipped with a constellation of beliefs, attitudes, dispositions, rules, convictions, fantasies, idiocies, hopes, plans and whatever. No two people, not even twins, have the same experiences and no two people have the same set of rules. However, these beliefs and rules are not all of the same nature or class. Some relate to the world, some relate to the self; some relate to the future and some to the past, some are mainly about emotional responses and some are about how to get things done. Because these rules are not the same, they cannot be classed on a single axis, or even on a dozen axes. Instead, they gel into loose but more or less independent clusters, just like plants and animals do, because that is their nature. These clusters are what the behaviorist questionnaires measure and these are what the biological psychiatrists hope will prove to have a genetic basis. It is possible there is a genetic factor in these clusters but it is indirect, not related to the nature of the beliefs themselves as it must work through another agency and, very often, that other agency is the innate cognitive system.

Ultimately, it is the innate cognitive system, which does have a genetic basis, which interacts with our experiences to determine our cognitive set on the world. The ICS determines whether a child will wilt under teasing or come out swinging. Teasing continues only when children don't stand up for themselves. The ICS determines whether a child will share or be selfish, will be cheerfully messy or prissily tidy, whether the child wants to spend more time with adults or playing with other children. This is not direct, the effect is indirect. The ICS determines only a tendency to react in certain ways as it is not a fixed response, such as insects show. The child's response to life events then biases the environment, slowly but subtly and powerfully reinforcing itself when those reinforcing events are unpleasant or, under favorable conditions, shifting the child's dispositions toward normal. Of course, each life event doesn't take place in a vacuum, it interacts with what has gone before, shifting the balances this way and that, depending on a myriad factors, some of which the individual knows and many he doesn't:

> Dr: "So why did you hit him?"
> Prisoner: "Nobody makes fun of my scar."
> Dr: "You got angry, but why did you get angry? Why didn't you keep quiet and let everybody see what a fool he is?"
> Pr: "I dunno, I just boiled up. It's been so many times, you got no idea. You think I'm tough but... (cries)."
> Dr: "But how can a scar reflect on the person underneath?"
> Pr: "Listen man, you got any scars? You got any idea what it's like?"
> Dr: "I've got something worse than a scar but I won't tell you if it will make you dislike me."
> Pr: "Yeah? I... I dunno, I never thought of it like that. I don't think that's what it is. They stare at me and whammo, I'm throwing

punches. Maybe I don't need to. It could be worse, couldn't it? Hey, doc, what about we swap chairs and you tell me all about it? Like, get it off your chest."

The behaviorist "model" of personality was not a model at all. It had nothing to do with internal causations of observable behavior but simply gave a crude measure of predictability of how a person would be likely to act based on how he thought he had mostly acted in the past. "Dispositions to act" are not things in themselves, they are not genes plugged directly in to the afferent motor tracts. We can characterize the individual's behavioral rules in English but it must not be forgotten that this is merely short-hand for a vastly complex system based in the brain structure. This system operates in a virtual space generated by information coded into particular neuronal systems. It is similar to the key shortcuts on a computer: "Ctrl-S means save." Underneath this convenient shorthand is a very fast, silent and hugely complex but perfectly rational set of operations which, *in toto*, save your work.

Some typical rules found in personality analysis include the following:

> Nobody tells me what to do.
> Don't make a fuss or draw attention to yourself.
> People will always try to cheat you.
> Most people will lend a hand if you ask them nicely.
> Never trust people in authority, they're out to get you.
> If you work hard and do the right thing, you will get your just reward.
> I'll never get a fair chance in life.
> Trust nobody.
> A place for everything and everything in its place.
> Disagreeing with somebody always causes offence.
> Always put others first.
> If people don't notice me, I'll die.
> If anybody looks at me, I'll die.
> If she talks to him, it means she's lost interest in me.
> Come what may, I have to be on time.
> That twinge means cancer.
> Live for today, tomorrow can look after itself.
> Anything I try will turn into a failure.

Underneath each of these convenient short-hands is a very fast, silent and hugely complex but perfectly rational set of operations which, *in toto*, determine how you act in the world. When all these injunctions are summated, we call that personality.

Because people learn their rules at different times and in different circumstances, there is no reason to believe they sit down later and rationalize what they believe. Contradictory rules may coexist, especially if they are context-bound. One rule may be activated in one set of circumstances and its complete contradiction may operate in another. In modern jargon, we could say: The outcome depends on the file path. One can readily see this in one's teenage children, who are rude, untidy, selfish and lazy at home but are unfailingly charming, winsome, considerate and helpful when they talk to adults other than their parents. Their behavior is context-bound as they wouldn't dream of being rude to their friend's parents. Similarly, without thinking objectively on what he is doing, the repressed gay man stares hungrily at the lifeguards marching past in their tight briefs but panics when he realizes somebody was watching him.

A potential objection to this approach is: How does the brain know which rules to activate? Answer: the brain doesn't, the mind does. There is a constant mental ferment of information entering the virtual realm, being sorted into significant items and dross, and activating a barrage of memories which then form the basis of behavior. This doesn't stop, even during sleep. In the deepest sleep, some rules are still active. I sleep soundly through the thunder of monsoonal rain pounding on an iron roof but will wake if a door creaks. Remember that the mind only needs give the briefest attention to a stimulus in order to activate a particular behavioral program, such as somebody brushing at a fly. If that split second of attention to the fly fails to enter memory, the action seems to have been unconscious. Everything is unconscious if you can't remember doing it. I walked up the stairs when I arrived home tonight but I have no recollection of stepping on the fifth step. That does not mean I did not intend it, it says only that the decision was not recorded in my memory as a separate event.

This is the cognitive basis of what Freud called ego mechanisms of defense. His model, it will be recalled, was non-scientific. He used the notion of a doorman standing in the door of a sitting room wherein consciousness was seated. Whenever objectionable guests came to the door, they were turned away by the doorman before consciousness had time to notice them. This is a pseudo-explanation, as it invokes a homunculus doing what requires explanation, thereby starting an infinite regress. It amounts to saying there are two different types of decisions, conscious and non-conscious but this is completely wrong. In effect, the psychoanalytic model equates conscious decisions with "those we approve of" and unconscious decisions with "those we don't."

The biocognitive model says that, in fact, all decisions are "unconscious" as we cannot introspect the actual decision-making processes themselves, and are only dimly aware, if at all, of the huge amount of information involved in those processes. I do not have to attend to the sequence of steps between an event and my response, all I have to do is focus on my goal and the cognitive processors of the mind do the rest. For example, I do not have to attend to my ciliary muscles when I focus close; all I do is "want" to look at my finger and the brain's data processing capacity relaxes the lens and the finger comes into focus. The process in my head is the same process as when chimps decide to groom their neighbors for fleas.

Of course, there are many levels of complexity between looking at my fingertip and finding reasons to justify my refusal to help when my enemy is in trouble, but the basic informational processes are the same. Incoming information is sorted and classified, then interacts with various standing instructions, beliefs, rules etc. so that a decision is computed and sent to the effector organs. Many of these rules are barely accessible to introspection, if at all, and the whole process takes place more or less instantaneously. It does not require anything like conscious intervention; quite often, decisions are not improved by attempting to "analyze" them too closely.

Any decision of mine which would normally be attributed to an "ego mechanism of defense" is qualitatively no different from a decision for which I wish to take full responsibility. It is the case that I have no access to the mechanism by which I make any decision; therefore, there is no conceptual difference between a decision I like and one I may have cause to regret, or one which "spares my feelings." Nobody makes a decision that, at the time, he believes is wrong decision to make. We may realize after that it was mistaken but we do not normally do anything that we believe at the time is morally wrong. Sure, I can justify to myself keeping the extra change a shopkeeper mistakenly gave me or but that is quite different from making a decision that suits me even though I know you won't like it. So I make a decision but then I immediately have to justify it to you, and this is when it gets embarrassing. There are no ego defenses from ourselves; they only come into play when I have to justify my actions to you. And "they" are nothing other than the same processes of normal decisions, compounded by the need to avoid looking foolish. The gay man watching the surf parade would be quite happy to indulge himself at home, watching it on TV, but it is different if he feels anybody is watching him. I may pick my nose in the privacy of my study, but not while meeting the bank manager.

Freudians split human decisions in two groups, the justifiable and the unjustifiable. They labeled the justifiable conscious and the unjustifiable unconscious, because that is what the patients and the analysts wanted. The biocognitive model says all decisions are the same. Strictly speaking, all decisions occur outside awareness although we know some or most of the information that contributes to the decision. To a classic Freudian, the reasons we make a prohibited decision are and always remain unconscious; they cannot enter consciousness because they would cause overwhelming anxiety. However, one of Freud's early, self-proclaimed disciples, Wilhelm Stekel [4], was of the view that it is not so much that we cannot see as we do not want to see. Freud, he said, used the analogy of torticollis whereby, by processes over which he has no control, the person's head is turned away from what might trouble him. Instead, Stekel used to term "scotoma," or blind-spot, to describe the process whereby a person conveniently fails to see what is obvious to everybody else. Stekel, who was influenced by Adlerian notions and later fell out with Freud, was of the view that the patient knows what it is he doesn't want to know: "I no longer believe in the overwhelming significance of the unconscious," he said. His insight was remarkable: we can hold any information we like in full consciousness, as long as it doesn't trouble us. That is, we have a choice over whether we feel bad about something, because knowledge and emotion are different cognitive elements. Information triggers emotion; if we don't like the emotion, we can still entertain the knowledge as long as we don't let it activate the emotional response:

> "Me? Ogling those lifesavers? Oh no, not at all, I was just inspecting their muscle development. A wonderful thing, muscle development, I had an uncle, you know, he'd been in the navy, taught me a great deal

about muscle development. He said a well-developed musculature is a sign of a strong personality. That's it, a strong personality. He had an extensive collection of pictures of well-developed—I mean, men with strong personalities. I admire that in a man and—oh, just look at the time. Have to hurry off, lovely meeting you."

When it comes to the important things, every one of us knows what we are about, all the time, even though we may have trouble stomaching the reasons in public. In some senses, it's almost a pity psychiatrists have to surrender the notion of unconscious causation. It made a great story and it meant the psychiatrist was never wrong, not to mention the money it generated.

10-4. Normal Personality

There is no such thing as a normal personality. The number of rules exerting control over our behavior is enormous, and all we could hope to do is discover the most important clusters of rules, rather than all the individual rules themselves. A set of rules which allows a person to lead a peaceful, productive life, in relative harmony with the surroundings, physical, social and cultural (and financial), amounts to a normal personality. It is clear there can be many different versions of the "normal personality," just as there can be many different versions of a normal face or a normal house. Of course, the definition of normal will vary from one culture to another, and one setting to another, but one of the crucial features of a normal personality in any setting is adaptability. The normal personality is able to adapt to abnormal circumstances such as illness, prison, war, disaster or major losses whereas the disordered personality soon comes into conflict of one form or another. Following great upheaval, during which desperate needs may compel desperate measures in order to survive, the normal personality will, normally, return to normality. Many don't.

People subject to major distress become different people, seeing the world through different eyes and reacting in ways they may not like. The person acquires new rules which may suit the bizarre new circumstances but afterwards, not everybody can rectify those changes. Henceforth, the unfortunate subject comes into conflict with the surroundings, shows disturbed behavior and experiences a wide range of mental symptoms. This is because the normal, harmonious adaptation to reality, both in the self and the surroundings, has been disrupted. This is not an illness in any physical sense of the word, but is a traumatically-induced change of personality.

It is important to remember that normality is a range, not a fixed point. People have good times and bad, they win some and lose some. They are happy when they win and sad when they lose, but normal sadness is not an illness, it is a genetically-determined response to a particular class of events which cannot be denied [5]. Normal people get angry at times or frightened at others, they may come into conflict with the law or abuse drugs or alcohol for a while but, crucially, they always go back to normal. People who habitually operate at the extremes are, by definition, not normal, and this means good people and bad. The highly successful in any field are as far from normal as the social casualties. Presidents and prime ministers, top academics and businessmen, intellectuals, sportsmen and entertainers, are not normal.

Normal people can't be bothered with the demands and dramas of getting to the top, they would rather spend their weekends taking their children to sport than attending meetings in distant cities. This is why great revolutionary leaders rarely make the transition to civil rule. Anybody who obsessively pursues a goal to the exclusion of a normal life, such as revolutionaries and crusaders, is not normal, not excluding psychiatrists who want to revolutionize psychiatry.

10-5. Abnormal Personality

The biocognitive model leads directly to a dimensional model of personality. The DSM-IV approach, which lumps personality disorder into categories, is completely wrong. It entirely misses the point of personality as the *generative mechanism* of observable behavior. There are no categories of personality disorder, unless the clinician stands so far away from the subject that the subtleties are no longer visible. The urge to find the Big Three Personality Factors (e.g. Eysenck), or the Big Five, or 200, is not empirically driven, but by ideological imperatives. The empirical fact is that any single human behavior distributes according to a normal curve. Therefore, any attempt to define cut-off points is arbitrary, not empirical; and since it is not empirical, it is not scientific. Because of this crucial point, an entire field of modern psychiatry is nonscientific which, of course, everybody knows but nobody will admit in public.

Because the question of personality disorder is so large, I will restrict this chapter to two aspects: (i) The failure of orthodox psychiatry to recognize anxiety as a personality factor; and (ii) the consequences of misdiagnosing personality disorder as mental illness.

10-5 (a). Anxiety as a personality factor

Orthodox psychiatry sees anxiety as a mental illness in the classic sense of the term [6]. It is held to be the surface or visible manifestation of a specific, genetically-determined biochemical lesion. Recent research on anxiety includes such insights as:

> "Neuropeptide S-mediated control of fear expression and extinction: role of intercalated GABAergic neurons in the amygdala" (Jüngling K, Seidenbecher T, Sosulina L, Lesting J, Sangha S, Clark SD, Okamura N, Duangdao DM, Xu YL, Reinscheid RK, Pape HC).
>
> "Differential effects of tumor necrosis factor-alpha co-administered with amyloid beta-peptide (25-35) on memory function and hippocampal damage in rat" (Stepanichev M, Zdobnova I, Zarubenko I, Lazareva N, Gulyaeva NV).
>
> "Acquisition of a conditioned avoidance reflex and morphometric characteristics of the sensorimotor cortex in rats subjected to social deprivation in early ontogenesis" (Levshina IP, Pasikova NV, Shuikin NN).

Anybody surveying the psychiatric literature on anxiety could be forgiven for thinking that psychiatrists have more interest in terrorizing rats than in dealing with frightened humans. However, it isn't all chemistry. S. Soltysik and P. Jelen uncovered this gem: "In rats, sighs correlate with relief." What is of real interest is that all of this activity is financed by grants.

The question then arises: is there such a thing as normal anxiety? Granted it is unpleasant, but does this ubiquitous emotion have a role to play in the human mental economy or is it always a case of pathology? This can be answered very succinctly: anxiety is a normal part of human life with a vital role to play in preservation of the individual and thereby of the species.

All animals display some sort of avoidance response whose effect is to safeguard the animal from threats. Limpets tighten their grip on their rocks; worms try to dig into the soil; birds scatter at high speed; fish ditto; at a particular, gruff warning bark from their mothers, young pups run for the nearest dark hole; a frightened primate infant reaches for its mother; frightened mothers reach for their babies, while frightened men run around in circles and arm themselves. Without the capacity to respond to threats, we would not be here today.

Anxiety is the emotion experienced in response to the perception of a threat. Threats are always in the future, approaching or coming at the individual. They impel a specific adaptive response, either stand and fight or run away. Any modern person leading an ordinary life who experiences anxiety more than once a week, or who experiences anxiety in differing settings, is an anxious person. An anxious person responds to neutral events in the environment as though they were a threat. When compared with the objective threat, his anxiety response is triggered too often and too intensely, to the point of interfering significantly with the quality of life and daily performance.

Biological psychiatry states that the anxious person suffers agitation because of a specific biochemical disturbance of brain function. The brain is abnormal. The biocognitive model says the brain is perfectly normal but is being fooled into responding to harmless events due to cognitive misperceptions or misappraisals of those events. The fault lies at the cognitive level, meaning the level of information coded into the brain. That is, treatment should be directed at the thought content, not at the machinery subserving thought. People are anxious because of what they believe about the world, about themselves and about their place in the world. Orthodox psychiatry has utterly failed to understand this critical point. More precisely, a person who habitually responds to harmless events as though they were threats has acquired "organizing principles" or rules which impel him to classify the events as threats, which then activates the anxiety response. As soon as I perceive a threat, I react. I don't think about it, otherwise I might die.

Given the definition of personality outlined above, it follows that an anxious person is responding to the world at the level of his most fundamental beliefs and attitudes, i.e. his personality. Chronic anxiety just is a personality disorder, one which generates excessive anxiety in a healthy brain. Chronic anger just is a personality disorder, one which generates excessive and inappropriate anger in a healthy brain. Chronic sadness just is a personality disorder, one which generates excessive sadness in a healthy brain. So what?

10-5 (a). Misdiagnosing anxiety as a brain disease

The failure of the DSM-type orthodoxy to understand the crucial point that emotions are driven by the cognitive set has led to the bizarre search for the "biochemical lesion" of a disease which does not exist. This wastes money on the type of pointless research mentioned above but the practical effect is to re-label people with disturbed personalities as suffering illnesses, thereby pressuring them to take drugs. Drugs, of course, have no effect on personality but, rather than admit the diagnosis may be wrong, the standard response from orthodox psychiatry is to prescribe more drugs. As time goes by, more and more people are being prescribed long-term medication for disorders which are not illnesses and will not respond to drugs. This is particularly seen in two diagnostic categories, the ADD/ADHD group and the group of Bipolar Affective Disorders.

I don't propose to field reams of statistics to show that the numbers of diagnoses in these two categories are rising rapidly, even as the numbers of people diagnosed as having personality disorders is dropping, nor to show that the rates of consumption of drugs used in these diagnoses are rocketing. Those figures are freely available on the internet and are cause for major concern. They show that prescription rates for these classes of drugs do not follow standard distributions for recognized diseases. There is enormous variation from one country to the next, even adjoining countries, and within countries. Crossing the state line significantly affects the diagnostic rates, as does moving from one city to another, or from city to rural areas, from one socioeconomic class to another, from one race or one sex to another, even from one school to another. The pressure on parents to have their children diagnosed as suffering a biochemical disease of the brain is enormous, as is the pressure on medical practitioners to diagnose them and then treat with drugs. Something is seriously wrong. DSM-III was supposed to standardize the process of diagnosis but not by labeling everybody. That is, we have traded validity for reliability: doctors can be relied upon to diagnose Johnny and prescribe drugs after a brief assessment. All that is lacking is that subtle element called validity. Psychiatrists (and pediatricians and family practitioners) can be relied upon to diagnose people as mentally ill, but the diagnoses are not valid. A very substantial proportion of people who, as recently as twenty five years ago, would have been assessed as having a disordered personality are now classed as mentally ill, with all that that label signifies. In fact, I see a far more ominous consequence beside dulled brains and ruined lives but first, some cases to illustrate the point.

Case 10-1. Mr. LJ, aged 26yrs.

This single man was referred for assessment after he found some material on the internet: "Asperger's Syndrome," he cheerfully announced, "that's me." He was working as a storeman/ controller in an explosives warehouse in the mining industry and lived in shared accommodation. He complained of feeling terrible all the time. He slept poorly, had little interest or motivation in his work and did very little after hours but sit at his computer, playing long-term games on the internet. His memory was patchy but his concentration was "too good," meaning he could ignore people by focusing on tasks. Unless occupied, he daydreamed and often missed what was happening around him. He hated his work and weekdays were a torture but he felt very good on weekends, when he stayed up all night playing his games. What was the trouble at work? His hands were always sweaty, his heart pounded, his stomach churned and he often felt he would faint if anybody spoke to him. He had an extensive list of fears, including germs and contamination (he washed his hands dozens of times a day) but most of his fears were social in nature, concerned with his performance and how people would judge him. He felt strongly that people were likely to threaten him and he should avoid contact where possible. He arranged his belongings in complex patterns and hated anybody touching anything of his. He touched and counted things and arranged them in strict orders of color coding and numbers. He had been like this all his life but had had no treatment.

His family background was disturbed as his parents separated when he was very young and he had no further contact with his father. His mother lived only for her children. She had no social life of her own, no hobbies and no interests beyond what her children needed. His only brother was, he said, highly intelligent but worked only as a delivery driver and they rarely spoke. He had hated school. He was short, chubby and did not play sport. He was bullied so his mother kept changing his schools or taught him at home until, at fifteen, he was taken to a martial arts class by a relative and enjoyed it. The bullying stopped and he was much happier as he could go to the library and nobody bothered him. He made friends with some of the shyer girls but never went out with them. On leaving school, he had unskilled jobs for a few years, then began studying IT but never finished the course. He had had many jobs but always left because he didn't get on with the other men. He liked the explosives job as security was high and he could stay in the building all day and hardly see anybody. He had had one or two girlfriends but drifted apart from them.

He didn't see that he had a problem: "There's nothing wrong with me," he said, "it's them." He saw himself as nervous, unassertive, self-conscious and highly mistrustful of people. He held grudges, kept his temper to himself and avoided authority. His self-esteem was "terrible," as he felt a failure in some sense: "I'm different, people don't like that." The mental state showed a rather boyish chap in plain casual clothes carrying gaming magazines. He was rather distant and hesitant but fairly cheerful and inquisitive of the processes of psychiatry. He was clearly intelligent but educated below his abilities.

He was commenced on specific treatment for anxiety and, at the first review, said he was feeling very much better: "This is fantastic. So that's all it was, then, anxiety? Damn, I liked being a syndrome."

Case 10-1. Discussion.

This man met criteria for a number of different disorders: Asperger's Syndrome/Autism Spectrum Disorder; Obsessive-Compulsive Disorder; Dysthymic Disorder; Social Phobia; Panic Disorder; Avoidant Personality Disorder and, with a bit of a push, Schizotypal Personality Disorder. What does this mean? For a biological psychiatrist, the minimum number of entities or diagnoses capable of giving a full account of this man's problems is six, possibly seven. In the standard biological approach, it means he has a number of separate genetically-determined, biochemical disorders of the brain which manifest in odd behavior and unstable moods. Yet, in ordinary medical terms, this seems to violate the principle of least causation, better known as Occam's Razor, which says that the number of explanatory entities must not expand beyond the practical minimum. In biological psychiatry, the observations to be explained become the diagnoses; they have no explanatory power, so they can expand endlessly. At the same time, the number of potential genetic defects seems to be very, very large. The human genome codes for something like 25,000 proteins using some three billion DNA base pairs, so there is very considerable scope for genetic errors to affect the brain. For each diagnostic category, the number of explanatory entities is fixed at one. A single genetic defect provides a full explanatory account for each single diagnosis. How does this violate the notion of least causation? Obviously, it doesn't.

The problem does not lie within the model of biological reductionism as it is applied to psychiatry, but with the entire concept itself. That is, biological reductionism will always assign a single chemical defect to each diagnosis because that is what it is designed to do. Instead, the question is whether biological reductionism is the correct model in the first place. Is there some other model that can give a simpler explanation of this man's various problems without postulating an endlessly expanding number of lesions which we may never be able to identify? The search is for a single intervening variable which can give a full and economical account of his various disorders.

In the first place, the most economical approach to mental disorder is to remain wholly within the mental realm itself. This bypasses the ineffably complex question of how genetic defects work their effects upon the mental realm. Secondly, by dispensing with the notion of categories of mental disorder, replacing this model with the dimensional approach, we simplify the question hugely. Finally, all we need to do is find a single mental factor which can, directly or indirectly, generate the observable behavior which needs explanation. Of course, it is glaringly obvious: LJ is an anxious person. His cognitive set on the world and his place in it (which is wholly a mental construct) generates unbearable levels of anxiety (again, wholly mental) which makes his life a misery and drives him to make behavioral adaptations with the goal of minimizing his anxiety. So, by abolishing the dubious categorical system of diagnosis, we can develop a unitary explanatory entity which leaves his genome, and all its attendant problems, right out of it. It also incorporates his personal history which, strictly applied, biological psychiatry would ignore.

So, instead of saying that this man has six or seven separate biochemical disorders which were not caused by his life experiences, we can now say his early life experiences caused him to develop a personality structure which generates excessive anxiety which, in turn, causes him to lead an abnormal life as an adult. Moreover, the concept of the innate cognitive system, which almost certainly has some genetic basis, argues that his genetic endowment probably did influence his early life experiences which then caused him to act upon his social environment in such a way as to generate adverse consequences (negative reinforcement, in Skinnerian terms). That is, genetic endowment plus family life puts him in a vulnerable position in his early social life (school), which was very frightening (the bullying) leading to withdrawal (his innate response) and further isolation, thereby restricting his personal and social development during adolescence, leading him to withdraw into a fantasy world rather than endure the anxiety generated by interacting with people. The obsessionality is of no causative significance at all but is another manifestation of the recursive anxiety state. Treating the anxiety led to an immediate improvement in his functional level and his level of comfort.

I believe this represents a vast improvement on the biological model. It satisfies the requirements of an economical explanation, incorporates the biological endowment (intellect, innate cognitive system), takes account of his early longitudinal personal development and also offers a point of intervention: treat the anxiety. This was done and, in two outpatient appointments spread over a week, the quality of his life was dramatically improved. That, surely, is economical.

10-5 (b). ADD/ADHD and personality disorder.

Case 10-2. Mr. AT, aged 21yrs.

A. arrived in Darwin with a letter from a psychiatrist in another city (this means about 4000km away, as Australia's Northern Territory has only one rather small city). He was unemployed, had little money, knew nobody in town and had been living in his car since he arrived. In a few bland lines, the letter said that he had a long history of ADHD and had been prescribed large doses of dexamphetamine for several years.

From the moment he arrived in the office, his manner was pushy and demanding. He said he had only come for "his drugs" and he didn't see the need for giving his history as "his shrink" had already made the diagnosis and nobody in such a useless town as Darwin would know what he was doing, anyway. Swearing copiously, he described frequent bouts of intense agitation in the setting of a highly suspicious and resentful personality. He had an extensive list of fears, mostly social in nature, and also suffered fairly regular bouts of feeling low and hopeless.

His family background was severely disturbed. His parents had separated after many years of fighting and he had gone from one to the other with several periods in care. His older brothers had extensive criminal records. He had attended perhaps a dozen schools before finally being expelled at age fifteen for fighting. Since leaving school, he had had a few brief jobs but always walked out or was dismissed after arguing or fighting. He had had several girlfriends but each left him because of his aggressive behavior and uncontrollable jealousy. He had used a wide variety of drugs as well as drinking heavily and had a long record of trouble with the police, starting at about age twelve.

Physically, he was of average height but lean and muscular. He had numerous tattoos, studs and scars. His behavior fluctuated between a sneering disdain, sullen boredom and angry demands. He was irritable and suspicious, alternately manipulative and threatening, yet was clearly of well above average intelligence.

Finally tiring of this folderol, he slammed his fist on the desk: "So what do I have to do to get my f—g drugs?" he demanded angrily. "Smash your f...g face in?"

He was told that jealousy and suspicion were contraindications for amphetamines and that he did not reach local criteria for them anyway. He was offered alternative forms of management but he stormed out. Two days later, a telephone call from a doctor in a town some 2,000km away revealed that A. was calmly telling people I had prescribed amphetamines for him but he had lost them while hiking in a national park.

Case 10-2. Discussion.

Quite clearly, this is a typical case of psychopathic or antisocial personality disorder with paranoid traits. His paranoid beliefs triggered intense anxiety which he relieved in the time-honored way of getting into fights or taking drugs, or both. He liked amphetamines because they relieved the anxiety and left him feeling razor-sharp and in control. Because he was not very big, he was careful about getting into fights and much preferred the steely alertness of amphetamines to the sodden joys of alcohol. Amphetamines allowed him to choose his victim and the time and place of the fight whereas alcohol usually ended in him picking the wrong person and being thrashed.

My enquiries have revealed that the psychiatrist who diagnosed him as having ADHD is a mild-mannered old chap who sees a lot of aggressive young drug-users with criminal records who come from severely disturbed backgrounds. His procedure is to give the patient a questionnaire to complete in the waiting room, talk to him (occasionally her) for a few minutes, and then prescribe amphetamines. He then refers the "patient" back to his family doctor to continue the drugs and doesn't see him again until the mandatory review at twelve months. According to another patient, he charges heavily for this service.

This is just bad psychiatry but it is licensed by the biological-DSM approach. The problem with the ADD/ADHD diagnosis is that is selects a small group of symptoms common to a considerable number of diagnoses, elevating these to over-riding diagnostic importance while ignoring all other significant material. Once the diagnosis is made, there are very powerful pressures to keep it in place. For parents, the cause of their offspring's obstreperous behavior is forever settled, and it doesn't include bad parenting. For teachers, boisterous or otherwise difficult students can be rendered tractable. For schools, there is extra money for managing a student with a "disability" which is not available for mere behavior disorders. For the "sufferer," there is the inestimable convenience of being able to shift responsibility for bad behavior to his chemistry. He also gets drugs with an extremely high black market value, and the chance of a disability pension from age sixteen with no questions asked. A single psychiatrist who elects to take this tidal wave of pressure head on runs the risk of having more than just his face smashed in. Fortunately, not all people who acquire the diagnosis are so pleased with it.

Case 10-3. Mr. BT, aged 19yrs.

This young man was referred for psychiatric assessment after he applied to enlist in the defense forces. During his medical interview, he had mentioned he had been prescribed amphetamines at the age of fifteen. When he was seen for psychiatric assessment, he was working and was not taking any medication.

A detailed history and mental state examination showed no evidence of current mental symptoms. There was nothing of note in his family history. He came from a stable family background with both parents working in quite demanding, office-based careers which involved a lot of travel. He had attended private schools throughout. At the age of fifteen, when his father applied for an overseas contract, B. was sent to an interstate boarding school. He hated it but he was unable to convince his parents he should come home again. He recalls he lost interest in school and began playing up, annoying the other boys in the class or arguing with the teacher. Under pressure from the school, he was referred to a pediatrician who diagnosed ADD and prescribed dexamphetamine. B. hated the drugs as he felt they meant he was "mental." After the second term holiday, he solved the problem by refusing to get on the aircraft to go back to the school. He was offered home schooling through the state Education Dept. so he stopped the medication and studied at home with no supervision. At the end of the year, his results were good enough for him to be offered an apprenticeship even though he was still below the normal age.

Case 10-3. Discussion.

This young man did not have a personality disorder, but his management was no better for it. The pediatrician's case records were detailed and entirely medical/behavioral in their focus. There was no mention of the boy's unhappiness at the school. While it may have been good pediatrics, it was still bad psychiatry. Bad psychiatry doesn't prove that psychiatry is bad *per se,* just as having to eat tasteless food in schools and hospitals never convinced me to stop eating. However, when psychiatry is such that busy pediatricians think they can sort out lives in twenty minutes, one wonders why we need psychiatrists. The answer is that we need psychiatrists to write the DSM so everybody else can go home feeling they have done a good day's work. It is one thing for various disciplines to try to take over psychiatry's traditional fields, it is something else again for psychiatrists to give it away.

Case 10-4. Mr. MS, aged 29yrs.

M. arrived with a letter from an interstate psychiatrist saying he had been diagnosed as suffering Adult ADHD and was prescribed dexamphetamine SR and lamotrigine. Since his arrival in Darwin, he had worked as a rigger on a large construction site for about twelve months. He had been obtaining supplies of amphetamines from the interstate psychiatrist (which is highly illegal) but he had run out some months before. He complained of "bad mood swings, always angry and sorta depressed." He was always active and had to exercise every night in order to get to sleep. He enjoyed work as it kept his mind occupied and he was able to talk to the other men. Socially, he did not mix well: "Hard to talk, always awkward and really anxious." He said his memory and concentration were "terrible." He had always been a dreamer but he also described high distractibility. He had trouble thinking clearly, with difficulty focusing on tasks and his thought content was endlessly preoccupied with what might go wrong. His mood was "mostly down, hopeless and useless, sick of myself." He had occasional suicidal ideas. He suffered frequent bouts of intense agitation with many somatic symptoms of anxiety. His only relief was to get away by himself. He had an extensive list of fears, mainly social in nature, including threats, criticism, saying No to people or letting anybody down, making mistakes or failing at anything and of going crazy and losing control.

His family background was unsettled. His father was an old biker who was a hard-drinking, opinionated and abusive man who constantly belittled his son for any mistakes he made. He had lost contact with his father but kept in touch with his mother, who was a very mild person. His siblings were scattered and he had not spoken to them for years. At school, he was interested only in science and astronomy, a dreamer who wrote little novels in class. He was shy and had no confidence at sport. On leaving school, he studied IT at a technical college for about a year but could not concentrate. He lived at home and had very little social life. When he left the college, he started drifting around the state, taking unskilled work until he tried rigging to overcome his fear of heights. He never did, but he had an aptitude for the technical side of the work. Socially, he had had a number of unstable relationships but he was "jealous and paranoid" and they didn't last. He drank erratically, used no illegal drugs and had a minor police record.

He saw himself as "pretty low, a failure." He described himself as nervous, erratically assertive and bothered by guilt, shame and self-consciousness. He was highly mistrustful of people but feared loneliness. He was jealous, avoided company and held grudges. He was very tidy and organized but ignored rules if they were inconvenient but still managed to get on quite well with authority. He saw his temper as "pretty bad," his intellect as "above average" and his self-esteem as "hopeless, a loser." The mental state showed an anxious but intelligent, youthful man with no tattoos, studs, scars or jewelry. He showed no defect of attention or concentration and was of superior intellectual ability.

Specific treatment for his anxiety state resulted in a rapid improvement. He reduced his alcohol intake and was not using any other drugs.

Case 10-4. Discussion.

The DSM-tick-a-box approach to psychiatry assigns diagnostic significance to superficially observable behavior. However, asking superficial questions will yield a superficial assessment. If psychiatry is only a matter of handing people a questionnaire and then prescribing drugs based on their responses, then the whole thing can be printed on the back of cereal boxes for people to diagnose themselves at breakfast, and then collect their tablets on their way to school or work.

Psychiatrists must not only elicit the symptoms but also need to offer an explanation, in terms of a given theory, as to why those symptoms exist. For a committed biological psychiatrist, the answer is: "Brain chemicals." Brain chemicals directly and inevitably lead to the observable behavior and no more explanation is possible or necessary. Drugs will correct the biochemical anomaly such that the observable behavior will correct itself. To me, that is simplistic to the point of inanity. It is abundantly clear in this case that personality factors generated the emotional states which then drove his behavior in certain directions. It is the job of the psychiatrist to delineate these internal factors and their associated states so that the behavior can be precisely targeted and corrected. Anything less is not psychiatry.

For example, while at school, M was a dreamer. Boys can be dreamers because they are too shy to mix, or because they are bored senseless by the class routine, or because they have no interest in school and wish to leave to work, or because they hate the teacher, or because they are crippled by performance anxiety and can gain pleasure only through fantasy, and so on. Somewhere, there may be a case for boys being dreamers because of a chemical imbalance of the brain but I am unable to conceptualize what that might mean. It would, of course, be very valuable if we could find out exactly what it means because then we could manufacture the chemical involved and everybody could be a Proust. Strangely, dreamy girls are not seen as such a worry.

This case clearly illustrates the role of anxiety as a perturbing factor in mental life. It is the mediating factor driving a great deal of disturbed behavior, just because it is the only truly aversive innate human emotion of sensation. Pain, of course, is highly aversive but it is externally-applied. Any personality factor that produces anxiety will have a perturbing effect on goal-directed behavior. Unfortunately, there are so many factors capable of producing anxiety that we could never list them all. The problem is greatly compounded by the fact that anxiety can become its own stimulus, thereby setting up a self-reinforcing or vicious circle which takes control of the individual's behavior just because anxiety is so overwhelmingly powerful. This case also shows that it is not so much a matter of whether the individual is anxious (although that is terribly important) but what he or she does with it. M. could have taken to alcohol or opiates to control his anxiety, or joined a cult of mushroom-eaters, or become a withdrawn fantasist, or taken up serious violence, or used his obvious talents to hack computers. There are so many career paths open to the true panicker, but he became a rigger. This used many of his technical skills, kept him apart from the general public and allowed him to pretend he wasn't scared of heights. It also let him look down on people, which he much preferred to people looking down on him.

Case 10-5: Ms. PR, aged 28yrs.

This woman was referred from an isolated mining town for an opinion. She was living with her three children and her most recent partner, having moved from interstate a year before. She was taking valproate (Depacon) 1500mg per day, first prescribed by a psychiatrist years before. She said she had had "heaps" of drugs at different times but claimed she was allergic to all of them as they made her aggressive: "I'm Bipolar Affective Disorder roughly and I think I'm having an episode right now."

From the outset, her behavior was pushy and controlling. She described "shocking" disturbances of sleep, appetite, energy, activity, interest and motivation. Socially, she insisted she avoided people except she had "huge numbers" of friends in her home town. Her memory was excellent, her concentration "atrocious" except when driving and she had "too many thoughts, jumping around, going back and forth." She was low and miserable "60% of the time" but her moods changed rapidly, swinging in minutes from "real sick of life" to "extreme highs, on top of the world," depending on what was happening around her.

She had frequent bouts of agitation with many somatic symptoms of anxiety, perhaps half a dozen a day lasting half to one hour each. During these, she was "ferociously" angry and argued with anybody in range. These were caused by any minor upset "depending on my mood," by people looking at her and "the son with the ADHD, he can't stop." She had an extensive list of social fears and strong feelings of people looking at her and talking behind her back. She was "ferociously" tidy and organized and became angry if anybody made a mess. She was ritualistic but there were no true obsessive-compulsive features.

These symptoms had been present as long as she could recall. She had seen several psychiatrists after overdoses as a teenager and numerous psychologists: it seemed the first people she contacted in any new town were the welfare services.

Her family background was seriously disturbed. Her father was an "angry, vicious, violent drunk" while her mother was a "bad-tempered, nasty, lazy, alcoholic slut with schizophrenic tendencies." She had a younger half-brother who had "mental issues," meaning he had been in mental hospitals and was a "bipolar borderline with schizophrenic tendencies" who was maintained on depot antipsychotics. After the parents separated, her mother often left her at home with the brother while she went away with different men or when she was in hospital. There were many drunken brawls in the house over the years.

Despite the home environment, Ms. PR claimed she had done "brilliantly" at school and got on extremely well with the teachers and with the other children. She was not shy or nervous but was "very, very loud" and argued and fought all the time with the teachers and other children. She did not play sport. On leaving school at 15yrs, she started working in shops and quickly became pregnant. After the baby was born, she said she became the manager of a large supermarket, then "ran" the dementia wing at a large nursing home and had several other important jobs. She left jobs because she had "meltdowns from the stress" or had "spack attacks." She had two children by her first partner but left because of his drunken violence and jealousy. The next partner lasted long enough for her to get pregnant, then there were two brief liaisons before the latest, who had been with her about a year.

She saw herself as "a very good person and mother." She agreed she was very nervous and bothered by guilt and self-consciousness. She was highly assertive, to the point of arguing with anybody, especially authority. She claimed she was very trusting and loved company except when she needed to sort out her head space but was also very jealous and held grudges. She didn't see any need to follow rules and evaded the question of how she related to authority. Her temper "depended," she saw herself as "highly intelligent" but her self-esteem was poor: "Don't have any. What a weird question."

The mental state showed a dumpy, overweight woman in plain clothes with tattoos and studs. Her manner was loud, pushy, controlling and demanding. There were no psychotic features. She was clearly of above average intelligence but poorly educated. She argued over the meanings of words, disputed the significance of symptoms and continually reminded the interviewer she had been diagnosed by an expert but also kept up to date with psychiatry on the internet. She had researched everything there was to know about "Bipolar" although she thought she might be "Borderline" as well. For treatment, she suggested she needed to be "monitored" by a psychiatrist because she liked talking.

Case 10-5: Discussion.

With a history like this, a categorical diagnosis becomes an exercise in the interviewer's prejudice. She had so many symptoms that, depending on how the questions were asked, her complaints could match practically any standard diagnosis at all. Review of case notes from another hospital clearly indicated that this had happened. The assessment was a check-list completed by a nurse and simply confirmed by the medical officer who assigned a diagnosis, prescribed drugs after a cursory interview and signed the last page.

The point of this case is that her history *mimics* the manic-depressive or bipolar syndrome. The DSM-IV diagnosis of Bipolar Disorder is purely observational. It does not attempt to "look beneath the surface" of the patient's presenting behavior. In a biological psychiatry, this makes sense as all that lies beneath the surface manifestations of mental disorder is a biochemical disturbance of the brain, which nobody can see anyway. However, this also means that nobody can say whether a case is the pure syndrome or merely a copy. For example, a person may complain of being hot. In a biological model, this would be diagnosed as "Heat Disorder." It would not distinguish between a true fever, a person who has been exercising or some-body living in the tropics. The reason biological psychiatry cannot sort cases with the same clinical appearance into different groups, according to their mental causes, is because it does not recognize mental causes. DSM-IV, being avowedly non-etiological, groups cases without regard for causes which, of course, was the basis of the case against Depressive Disorder carefully assembled by Horwitz and Wakefield [5].

On the other hand, the biocognitive approach says that the final clinical picture is the result of innumerable mental mechanisms. The psychiatrist's job is to sort the surface symptoms and probe the underlying mental factors before assigning them their proper causative significance. This is a profoundly different approach to psychiatry. The current biological emphasis produces a psychiatry which lends itself, if not actually encourages, the notion that psychiatry is just a matter of a nurse ticking a few boxes, then ringing the medical officer to write a script for a patient who will come back for review in a month. At his review, the patient may see a different staff-member who will simply flick through the standardized intake checklist, ask a few questions and then write a further script. Psychiatry becomes a commodity, meaning "goods or services whose provenance is of no significance."

To illustrate the notion of a commodity, in the old days, when you bought tomatoes, you would go to a particular shop because the proprietor had better fruit. He would ask you what you liked, and then advise you what you should buy. You could choose from his grosse lisse or beefsteaks, romas or Russian blacks as the fancy took you. These days, however, when you buy a pound of tomatoes, you buy a commodity. No matter which shop you go to, you will get an absolutely standard pack of hard red balls from an industrial farm which have been picked green by mechanical pickers, then shipped through several time zones before being packed in plastic and dumped in a chilled display by staff who wouldn't know a tomato from a baseball unless it was written on the package. You cannot tell where your tomato came from, because it no longer matters. This has happened to computers, to cars, to clothes and now to medical services but for different reasons. In cardiology, we want services and procedures standardized because that is the only way to ensure a uniformly high standard. We do not want cardiologists in poor areas saying to their unwilling patients: "Good morning, I'm your cardiologist but, actually, I failed." Psychiatry, however, has gone the extra mile by dispensing with the psychiatrist as a "significant variable" in the relationship of patient to recovery. Treatment has been commoditized, homogenized and neutered to the point where the questionnaire is more important than the person who administers it. If there are only a certain number of boxes for the patients to fit in, it doesn't matter who hammers them in.

The biocognitive model, on the other hand, says the psychiatrist is of critical importance, the difference between a pilot bringing an airliner into land or the hostess. In Case 10-5, we start by looking at the behavior, meaning bouts of excitement alternating with despair, grandiosity, irritability and her generally disorganized life. We then look for the underlying causes of these features but the important part of this task is to sort the observable features into causes and effects. Thus, the physical symptoms of psychomotor agitation are classed as features of anxiety, not depression. Because anxiety is an emotion, it is a secondary phenomenon, not primary, and a cause must then be found for it. It will be found buried in the patient's rules or injunctions. This is totally different from the standard, DSM-IV approach, which does not look for causes. Anxiety, in that view, is a "stand-alone" phenomenon, it co-exists or is "comorbid" with depression. The biocognitive model says depression must also have a cause, and the commonest cause is an unsuspected anxiety state.

This woman shows why anxiety states are so often unsuspected: modern psychiatry is obsessed with depression—it dismisses anxiety as a minor nuisance—while patients are equally obsessed with not revealing their anxiety, which they see as a moral weakness. By this means, we reach the point of the intellectually blind leading the willfully unseeing. Under these circumstances, the drive to commoditize psychiatry becomes understandable, if not excusable.

Case 10-6: Ms. MA, aged 26yrs.

This single student was referred for assessment two weeks after she had arrived in Darwin from a southern city. She was staying in a backpackers' lodge was receiving an invalid pension for "bipolar." She had been seeing psychiatrists for years and was taking lithium 675mg per day, quetiapine 50mg at night and clonazepam 2mg at night. She had fled from her home in a state of panic, with no clear idea where she was going or why. She described feeling "very unsettled," with poor sleep, loss of appetite, low energy and activity and low interest and motivation. Socially, she was avoiding people and had no sexual interest at all. He concentration was poor and she had "too many thoughts spinning around" her head. She felt confused and unhappy but not as low as she had in the recent past.

The main finding was a severe anxiety state with frequent bouts of intense agitation lasting hours on end. She had an extensive list of fears, mostly social in nature, but no paranoid ideas. She was a fastidious person but there were no obsessive-compulsive features. These symptoms had been present for years but had not improved with extensive psychiatric treatment and she was finally granted a pension. She believed she had a chemical disturbance of the brain as well as "learned negative reactions to criticism." The psychotherapy was "Freudian-oriented and mindfulness" but she had had many forms of therapy in the past.

Her family background was unremarkable. Both her parents had responsible jobs but she described her mother as "compulsively depressed and PTSD" following an assault many years before. Her older brother worked in IT and was "calm and intensely hard-working." She did extremely well at school and won a scholarship to a prestigious private school, where she excelled in all her classes but her main interests were music and drama. She went straight to a very demanding course in music and theater, during which she moved in with one of her teachers for convenience. The teacher was renowned as domineering, demanding, highly critical and possessive, and Ms. A became increasingly anxious that she could not satisfy the older woman's expectations. Her mental state gradually deteriorated and she was eventually referred for treatment. After she graduated, she decided she should gain another degree, this time more socially beneficial. She became increasingly disorganized but struggled through the course with several admissions to hospital after overdoses. She had very little social life, drank very little and used no illegal drugs.

She saw herself as very concerned about other people's needs and socially responsible. She was anxious and unassertive and intensely bothered by guilt, shame and self-consciousness. She was rather wary of people but tried to keep the peace at all times. Socially, she used her acting training to give the impression of *savoir faire*. She saw her intellect as high and her self-esteem as very poor. The mental state showed a slim young woman who would pass for years younger, dressed in clean clothing with no tattoos, studs or jewelry. She was well-spoken, courteous, cooperative and keen to talk. She was rather weepy with no psychotic features and was clearly highly intelligent. She felt she needed treatment but had no idea what could benefit her as she had tried most of them. Soon after the initial assessment, she decided to return to her family and try to resume her studies.

Case 10-6: Discussion.

What is the relationship between mental disorder and personality? Orthodox psychiatry says there is no relationship, they are independent mental states which do not influence each other. This young woman clearly showed a cluster of personality traits which were not compatible with a happy life. She was socially anxious and greatly concerned with how people would see her and judge her, to the point of being incapable of saying "no" to anybody yet resentful if their demands prevented her pursuing her own goals. She suppressed her anger and deferred her own interests and ambitions in order to please everybody around her. These are clearly personality traits yet these factors contributed very substantially to her anxiety and her recurrent bouts of depression.

She also illustrates another important point. In general medicine, if a trial of treatment is unsuccessful, the physicians will try an alternative form of treatment. If this does not work, the diagnosis will be reviewed. If the treatment fails, reconsider the diagnosis. However, when a psychiatric patient fails to recover, the diagnosis is not questioned but the prognosis is revised downward: "It was such a tragic case. She had such wonderful promise but then she broke down and never really recovered." In this case, the reason she did not recover was because the pathological personality elements were not addressed. The conflict caused by her contradictory personal rules meant that she was always anxious and resentful, with occasional slides into frank depression when things were especially bad. Occasionally, if things went well or she was able to escape something particularly onerous, she would feel bright and cheerful for a day or two but it never survived the first upset. Again, she mimicked the bipolar or manic-depressive cycle but the cause was personality factors, not aberrant brain chemistry.

10-6: Conclusion.

In their search for rock-solid reliability, DSM-III and -IV dispensed with mental factors on the basis that they were inherently unreliable. This is a problem because, if the causes of mental disorder are mental factors, then biological psychiatry throws the baby out with the bathwater. A person may be socially withdrawn because he believes he is inferior, or he fears assault, or he believes he smells, or he believes he will make a fool of himself, or he has bad teeth as he fears dentists, or he might catch something, or he is so slow due to rituals that the party is over before he gets there. There is no limit to the reasons. However, the DSM committees still had to offer something as an explanation: if we can discern different surface syndromes, there must be deeper underlying causes, so they opted for the ultimate "underlying cause," genetics. Nobody could argue with that, nobody could prove it wrong. That is a tragedy for psychiatry as it means that their ambition to prevent bad psychiatry is now strangling psychiatry. If nurses and psychologists and, nowadays, computers [6], can practice psychiatry, who needs a shrink? The patients do, that's who.

The surface picture of mental disorder is finite; the underlying mental causes are close to infinite. If the biocognitive model has a "take-home" message, it is this: "Look for the mental causes, because they are always there." If the diagnosis is wrong, the treatment will never be successful. If personality factors are producing the surface picture of mental disorder, but they are not addressed, then the patient will never get better because, by definition, personality doesn't change. This is why mental disorder seems to have such a poor prognosis, and drug companies can argue that mentally-ill people should take medication for life. Unfortunately, orthodox psychiatry slips easily into the trap of believing this line, but if psychiatrists were taught how to take a history these days, the prognosis for mental disorder wouldn't be so uniformly gloomy.

11

Circus Vitiosus

"Genuine progress means the continuous destruction of myths."
George Orwell, Collected Essays 1945-50

11-1. Introduction

In these busy modern times, where the pressure is on to *deal* with problems rather than waste time in idle contemplation of causes, it helps to have a little catchphrase or sound bite that pithily summarizes the guts of what we are about. As they rush off to their laboratories, biological psychiatrists can call over their shoulders, "Chemical imbalance of the brain," secure in the idea that it captures the urgency of their mission. Psycho-analysts were not renowned for doing anything in a sentence when they could have written a book about it (and had a schism), but "Id impulses breaking through" was enough to strike terror into the hearts of their clients. For behaviorists, we have to search a bit further, but our reward is in JB Watson's startling claim to be able to transform any infant into any adult: "Give me your little Johnny," he didn't quite say, "and I guarantee to train him to become any specialist you want, or a thief, regardless of his talents, tendencies, vocations or race" [1, p82]. On the far side of the behaviorist paddock, Skinner's brave new world of Walden Two was perhaps summarized by the idea of "Control and prediction of behavior." Skinner's vision of a world trimmed of all the fiddly bits (such as freedom and dignity), where all behavior is "shaped and maintained by operant conditioning" toward a centrally-planned goal, laid bare his ultimate ambition. Even for quibblers, the last line in *Beyond Freedom and Dignity* [2] clears up any doubts: "We have not yet seen," he trumpeted, "what man can make of man."

Really? Having seen the hash man has recently made of man's economy, how many of us would want to?

Just to settle the point, imagine, if you will, the first meeting of the Ethical Directions Committee of the new Supranational Commission for the Scientific Control and Prediction of Behavior. Mr. Gordon Brown, who, as Chancellor and later Prime Minister of the United Kingdom, brought the country to its economic knees, something two world wars didn't do, sits beside Mr. Christopher Cox, former Chairman of the US Securities and Exchange Commission, who failed to detect Bernard Madoff's activities despite ten years of warnings; they are joined by Mr. Rick Wagoner, former chairman of General Motors who gave you the Hummer in the midst of the global warming crisis, and Mr. Vladimir Putin, pre-eminent *eminence grise* of Russia, appointed for his unrivalled expertise in controlling everybody. In their deliberations, these civic-minded gentlemen are assisted by Governor Sarah Palin and Ms. Victoria Beckham from the newly-established Committee for Cultural and Esthetic Improvement. And for his unerring ability to forge ahead where lesser men pause for thought, the chairman could only be... (drumroll)... Mr. George W Bush.

On second thoughts, perhaps we might steal past Skinner's dystopian vision and leave it quietly gathering dust on the shelves.

In the face of such uplifting historical examples, I am afraid the biocognitive model flounders a little. To my keen regret, this is not a manifesto to inspire people to fling down their tools and rush into the streets to proclaim the millennium. National Logic Gates Day? It hardly quickens the pulse. So, aware of my duty to lunch-time television, I have pondered a suitable sound-bite although, to be perfectly transparent about it, nobody in the television industry, lunchtime or any time, has yet asked for my assistance, but I am ready. So here it is, my soundbite to swell hearts: *Circus vitiosus.* It has, readers will appreciate, a subtle flavor (full-bodied, with hints of classic sardonic humor over an astringent modern darkness) although there will, of course, be the usual disputes over pronunciation.

In my catchphrase, *Circus* has nothing direct to do with clowns or beefy ladies in tights cracking whips at little dogs; it just means ring or circle. *Vitiosus* means nasty, horrid or savage; thus, in English, a vicious circle. Let us, then, joyously shout *Circus vitiosus* from the rooftops before, somewhat embarrassed by curious stares from the passersby, we clamber down, muttering to each other: "So tell me again what it actually means?"

11-2. Homeostasis

We take our minds for granted. Actually, we take the entire miracle of the human body for granted as well, daily abusing it with rich food, drugs and alcohol, pollution, fast cars and discos, but the mind is not just a physical machine. Structurally, the brain is the most complex thing in the known universe. It has layers upon layers of complexity that we are only beginning to appreciate. Inevitably, this means the mind, the brain's actual function, is orders of magnitude more complex still. In talking of the mind, we are so accustomed to almost instantaneous recall of minor events from years ago that we rarely give a moment's thought to the prodigious feats of organization that must be involved in simply knowing where the memory is stored. Of course, I don't know where my memories are stored, only my brain does. I don't even know whether I have a brain.

It is, however, critically important to understand the nature of the dynamic balances that sustain mental life. Starting with the body, we are aware of the hugely complex modes of interaction of the many different systems that interact every second of the day, from the moment of conception to the moment of death. The human body works only within very narrow limits of function even though the body's owner may submit it to extremes of temperature or chemical and physical abuse. In addition, every living human is under constant assault by a huge range of microorganisms which, unless destroyed, could reduce the body to stinking pulp in minutes. The whole, vastly complex process of staying alive in a hostile environment was summarized by Cannon's concept of homeostasis, the notion that large numbers of self-correcting individual systems work together in a finely-tuned balance to maintain the internal milieu precisely within optimal levels of function.

It is essential to be fully aware of the nature of a living body as a constellation of finely tuned, dynamically-interacting controlled systems. The body is not like a house which, once built, simply stays in the same state while activity takes place in its rooms. It is not like a fire, sedately burning its quota of fuel then quietly fading away. It has to be understood as a system of, for example, spinning tops balanced on top of each other, with each top counteracting the action of its neighbors above and below. While the system is humming with energy, it is nonetheless in perfect balance and will stay in balance unless something happens to disturb one of its components. Then it will fly apart. Think of a jet engine slung beneath the wing of an airliner flying far above the clouds. To a passenger gazing idly out a window, the jet pod appears to be doing nothing much. Yet inside its nacelle, the turbine is spinning at many thousand rpm, with its hundreds of blades operating at white hot temperatures. As long as air is sucked into it and the fuel is available, it will continue to operate. However, if something hits one of the blades and unbalances it, the engine will explode in a shower of shrapnel.

That is roughly how the human body should be conceptualized. It is a vastly complex machine comprised of many subunits, where each and every element is in a state of high tensile, dynamic balance with every other part. A change in one element quickly induces changes in others, with the effects gradually moving through the entire system like ripples, until a new dynamic balance is achieved. It is a modification of le Chatelier's Principle: If anything disturbs a system in dynamic balance, then the balance will change in such a way as to negate the effects of the disturbance. The air temperature goes up, so the blood vessels in my skin dilate to lose heat. The air temperature goes down, so they constrict, then flow in the deeper peripheral blood vessels slows, then I start to shiver, and so on. All of this is part of normal physiology, which we take for granted just because it is so effective. But watching my hand at rest is rather like looking at the jet engine from the safety of my seat in the plane: looks pretty quiet out there, but things could go wrong awfully fast.

Our physiology is effective for two reasons. In the first place, it is breathtakingly complex. Even a brief look at the immune system shows the staggering complexity of this essential system [3] which is absolutely typical of our growing understanding of molecular physiology [4]. Secondly, the body is robust by virtue of very high levels of duplication and redundancy and because, when necessary, the many subsystems can operate in relative isolation. An infection in one finger activates the immune system which isolates the invasion so that it does not spread through the body. It is true that some parts of the body are more stable than others. For example, skin can survive hours without oxygen, whereas cardiac muscle is damaged beyond repair in a minute. Cerebral physiology in particular is extremely finely balanced, to the point where it can be profoundly impacted by events that would hardly be noticed by cells in another tissue. If the blood temperature rises or falls more than a few degrees or the CO_2 level rises a few percent, the brain begins to malfunction.

In normal daily life, the body functions within very narrow limits of tolerance. Any variation in one of many thousands of physical or chemical parameters will quickly trigger a corrective response. In order for this to happen, there are huge numbers of sensing systems which detect even minute changes from normality. Within the human body, many hundreds of physical control systems are known, and new ones are regularly discovered. Each of these widely dispersed control systems has three components: a receptor, which detects variations in the parameter; a control center; and an effector organ. The detectors are highly specific and highly sensitive: some can respond to a change in a hormonal level of just one part in a hundred million. This information is sent to a suitable dedicated processor which in turn activates the responder organ. These systems operate in the physicochemical realm and are governed by the laws of thermodynamics. They work just as well in sleep or anesthesia as in waking life, as there is no mental intervention at all (and certainly no homunculus or *elan vital*).

Whenever we look at a living person, even somebody in a deep sleep, we should see not a passive lump of meat but a highly organized, extremely delicate instrument made of many hundreds of subsystems. These work ceaselessly in concert to produce behavior which fits almost perfectly with the environment to achieve the body's ends. Watching somebody running, or playing the piano, or telling a joke while peeling a potato, is to see something astounding, so astounding that it may not exist anywhere else in our galaxy, if not further. Why anybody would think fantasy novels are more exciting than this is beyond me.

11-3. *Homeostasis Mentalis*

The behavioral complexity of the human body emerges from the finely-tuned and vastly complex interplay of many subsystems. Working in harmonious interdependence, these account for observable behavior without invoking non-material forces or entities. Every action and function is assembled from less complex elements, where the contribution of each subsystem can be derived by analysis of the final, emergent behavior or function. The body is not passive or inert but is in a state of ceaseless physicochemical activity which consumes energy and nutrients in order to maintain the steady state. This is what homeostasis means: self-maintaining stability.

The mind must be seen as another hugely complex homeostatic system. It differs only in the respect that it is not a physicochemical entity, meaning it is not governed by the laws of thermodynamics. "Mind" is composed of many subroutines interacting according to its own laws of logical systems such that observable behavior is assembled in a perfectly explicable sequence from basic elements. The whole entity is balanced and operates as a self-correcting and self-sustaining virtual machine. Putting aside the fact that it doesn't exist in the material world, this virtual machine is constrained by homeostatic principles analogous to those governing the physical body. This notion is critical to the understanding of the mind as a biocognitive virtual machine and especially to its disorders.

The most basic element in the development and function of mental life is the level of arousal. In Chap. 14 of my previous book, I placed great emphasis on the Yerkes-Dodson principle, the notion that there is an optimal level of arousal for any behavioral function, outside which performance deteriorates. Arousal is governed from above; in effect, the mind chooses how fast it wants to function, depending on the demands it perceives around it. In quiet surroundings, with no particular demands or pressures, the arousal level drops and the person starts to feel sleepy. Suddenly, he thinks he hears the boss coming. In an instant, he is alert and jumps into action. However, the footsteps keep going and he hears a car drive away; presently, his eyelids are drooping, his breathing is slowing and his mind is drifting away from the job on his desk. A person in a state of low arousal cannot focus on a specific task. However, a frightened person will find his mind spinning so fast he may have trouble keeping his mind on the problem. His mind is flooded with possibilities of how to deal with the problem that has startled him. That is, the threat raises his arousal, which causes his mind to throw up suggestions on how to resolve the threat; he then acts on one, the threat abates and he slips back into his resting state. This is Le Chatelier's principle at work: a system is in balance (worker dozing at his desk after lunch); something acts to alter the balance (footsteps in the corridor), so the system changes to negate the change (pretends to be busy). When the threat disappears, the system goes back to normal (leans back and closes his eyes).

Again, this is so normal in our daily experience that we hardly notice it but it is a core element of the model of the mind as an active, self-controlling system. This small example is important because it shows how the mind activates the brain in order to change its own function. That is, it depends on a precise (meaning molecular) solution to the mind-body problem. If there were not direct paths linking mental function to the arousal systems of the ascending reticular activating system (ARAS), then we would never be able to respond to perceived threats. Perception is a mental phenomenon and the behavioral response is physical: at some point, these two realms have to be joined. The entire glory of human intellectual achievement is utterly dependent on a nexus of relatively few neurons connecting the thinking, perceiving part of the mind to the activating part of the brain. Without that link, we would all be dead. Even when those links are only damaged, as in brainstem infarctions, the person is trapped, unable to talk or move.

Mental homeostasis differs from the physical model in that the mind does not act directly upon itself to produce arousal. In a physical machine, self-control is exerted by subsystems which function wholly in the physical realm. They may have a data-processing capacity, but this supplements or improves their function without being an essential part of it. There are plenty of control systems in my house and in my car which are purely mechanical. The carburetor on a real car was a good example of a very subtle control system with no digital processing ability whatsoever. In the mind, however, the control system begins in the physical realm (say at the level of the retina or cutaneous sensation), crosses to the mental, then loops back through the physical realm again in order to activate itself. This isn't always true; some mental control systems stay entirely within the mental realm, but they are not so central to mental life as the systems governing arousal.

A threat is perceived but, until the entire brain and then the body are activated, nothing happens. A threat is not a threat until I respond to it *as though* it were a threat. Otherwise, I would be no more agitated by it than I am by the crickets chirruping outside my window: "Fancy that, here comes that man with the gun again. That's a nice shirt he's wearing." Events are judged threatening by the cognitive section of the mind, drawing on a range of information from current input, memory and the innate cognitive system, then the instruction "Come to full arousal" is sent to the brainstem (not in English, of course). This signal activates the ARAS, which then activates the whole body, including the brain, readying it for fight or flight. This is a hugely complex matter which, unfortunately, hasn't received the attention it should from psychiatry. Orthodox psychiatry has been so preoccupied with finding a single chemical (now a gene) to account for over-arousal that it has completely missed the point: arousal is a normal response in an intact organism which affects every part of the body. There is only one sort of arousal, the jittery type. If a soldier in combat is not deemed to be in a disease state, then there is no reason to suppose that a person who fears giving a lecture is in a disease state: inappropriate, yes, even self-damaging, but not diseased.

In normal life, the mental realm functions as a seamless whole but it is actually composed of various subroutines which smoothly support each other. As I walk through the garden, different sights and sounds trigger memories, but these are appropriate to the setting. At normal levels of arousal, I am not bothered by irrelevant memories which distract me from my task; my mind ambles blithely from one topic to another and I simply go along for the ride. As this idle soliloquy unfolds, I derive a sense of continuity which, combined with my core beliefs, my likes and dislikes, memories, hopes and ambitions, amounts to me. There is no Self or I or field of consciousness separate from the interdigitating subroutines; what I call "I" is no more than a short-hand for "all that happens to be me."

Normal mental life maintains a balance between narrow limits, the same as normal physiology. In my garden are some new trees I have grown from seed. Each day, I like to see how they are growing. One morning, I find one of them wilting, and a quick jerk on the stem shows it has been chewed off underground, per courtesy of *Mastotermes darwiniensis*, the Godzilla of termites. Rather than flying into an impotent rage against termites, I quickly decide to spray the remaining seedlings and buy some more seeds to try again. Without explicitly thinking of the full range of my options, I have maintained my mental balance by adapting to reality. Equanimity is the goal of gardeners. Football fans are different. Their only goal is victory over the competition. If their team goes down, they slink home a bit glum but, after a few beers, they feel better because, without admitting it, they just know there's always next week. We cannot remain in an unsettled mental state for long, something has to change and this process of restoring balance is automatic. I do not have to run through the different scenarios to come to the conclusion "Let this seedling go, there will be more." It would take a lot of defeats before a football fan reached the point of changing teams but it will happen. In politics or religion, a person may preserve his equanimity by choosing "death before dishonor," but he will go to his death calmly. We have to preserve our mental balance.

We adapt to the world by a process of high speed computation of the options, where each option is weighted by processes we cannot introspect. We are not aware of the processes by which we reach our conclusions, we are merely apprised of the outcome. People are compelled to maintain their mental balance, and will twist and turn in their attempts to do so but are not aware of the steps they take. This is the basis of the Freudian notion of "ego mechanisms of defense." Without deliberating on it, we know perfectly well what will hurt us, so we keep right away from it. It is not the case, as Freudians claimed, that we cannot know what is repressed; rather, it is repressed because we are aware of what is we don't want to acknowledge. Ego defenses are simply *homeostasis mentalis* in action.

11-4. When Stasis Fails

11-4 (a) Stable instability

The idea of a self-maintaining mental stability is not new. Freudian and post-Freudian notions of ego psychology assumed a great deal of what homeostasis makes explicit. However, the advantage of rendering the concepts explicit lies in its value in explaining certain critical features of mental disorder. The principals on which the homeostatic biocognitive model of mind is built give rise to a novel approach to mental disorder as self-perpetuating mental instability. This follows directly from the idea of the mind as a vastly complex system trying to maintain its own stability in the face of ever-changing circumstances. For any complex machine, if the control mechanisms themselves slip into an abnormal state, then the mental balance will be lost but, most importantly, it will not be able to correct itself.

When we look at the central principle behind behaviorist, biological and early psychoanalytic concepts of mental disorder, we find it is the same in each case. Each one assumes that the cause of the mental disorder remains active until rectified. That is, they are based on a simplistic concept of mental disorder flowing inevitably from a static or persisting cause. To use a simple analogy, if I tread on a sharp spine, then the discomfort will continue unchanged until I remove the spine. This is also true of chronic disorders, such as diabetes. Here, the pancreatic islet cells fail to secrete insulin, and the disease persists until the problem is rectified, either by insulin supplements or by oral hypoglycemics. A continuing disorder implies a continuing cause.

Each of the old models of mental disorder, behaviorist, biological and early psychoanalytic, relies on the same concept. While it is not entirely fair to talk about behaviorist models of mental disorder, as they have largely faded from view, they are still used to supplement the dominant biological approach when convenient [5]. To a committed behaviorist, the core element, "wrong learning," will persist intact until it is rectified by "new learning." Whatever it is that is learned will continue to exert its effect until it is switched off, as it were. This is also true of the classic psychoanalytic model, in which the damaging factor, say, a forbidden id impulse, continues to try to break into consciousness until it is neutralized. At the other end, destructive superego prohibitions will remain active until replaced by more appropriate rules.

This notion is central to modern biological psychiatry. In this model, the cause of mental disorder just is a biochemical lesion, of some sort, in some part of the brain. Most authors accept that the lesion is itself caused by genetic faults although some give credence to the idea that experience can cause permanent changes to the brain. Either way, the significance of the lesion is that it is just that: a lesion. It is a fault, a biochemical sore, as it were, which exerts its effect as long as it is present. This is the corollary of the essential biological principle, that there cannot be a mental disorder unless there is a preceding biochemical fault. You can't have one without the other because the arrow of causation goes from brain to mind only: the converse is that mental disorder invariably implies a pre-existing biochemical disorder. The mental disorder will persist until the biochemical disorder is rectified, unless it rectifies itself which, being genetic, isn't likely. By the same principle, diabetes is not self-correcting and the spine in my foot isn't going to pull itself out. So far, so medical.

Medicine, however, has moved ahead of this simple model of direct causation, to take account of the body's many feedback mechanisms. There is now no dispute with the idea that, while homeostasis is critical to our survival, the mechanisms which support it can "get it wrong." That is, there are diseases which result not from an extrinsic cause but from a failure of intrinsic self-regulation. The large group of autoimmune disorders such as SLE and rheumatoid arthritis, and allergic disorders such as asthma, hay fever, and so on, are the result of errors of self-regulation rather than being continuing reactions to persisting causes. For whatever reason, the self-regulatory mechanisms become locked in an over-active state, thereby inducing a state of *dis-ease* which has no extrinsic cause. The attempts to rectify the fault in the internal milieu constitute the disease.

The biocognitive model of mental disorder relies heavily on this concept, that there is a (large) class of mental disorders resulting from errors of mental self-regulation, meaning they have no primary, extrinsic cause. It also allows the possibility that there may once have been an extrinsic cause, but the mental reaction has lost contact with this cause and has become self-perpetuating. This notion is diametrically opposed to the central element of biological psychiatry. It gives substance to the argument (Chap.2) that, in any self-regulating machine, a physical disorder can always be mimicked by a programming fault. It should be clearly understood that talk of "errors of self-regulation" does not imply a biochemical error. The homeostatic mechanisms are actually doing their job, but they are accidentally maintaining the mind in an abnormal state. That is, people can become locked in a self-perpetuating mental disorder which persists long after the original cause, if any, has completely faded.

11-4 (b). Panic states

The phobias are a clearly defined example of self-regulation gone awry. For whatever reason (including the innate cognitive system), a person develops a fear of frogs. Because the frog is now seen as a threat, i.e. he evokes the same response as a large and angry dog, the person reacts accordingly, he pulls away. Thus, his fear state fades, which is exactly how the fear reaction works: it compels the person to remove himself from the threat, and it doesn't fade until he does. The fear response is an innate, self-regulating reaction to perceived threats in the environment. It functions to protect the individual (person or rat) from danger. But frogs are not dangerous, so why does the fear reaction persist and intensify to the point where we say it is a disorder? It happens because the self-regulatory cycle of *perception of threat—fear response—withdrawal* "slips a cog," as it were. The person becomes more frightened of his own fear response than of the frog, although he normally won't be able to tell them apart. People do not normally distinguish between the actual threat of an event and their response to it: to most people, they are one and the same thing. A person with a fear of snakes will not normally distinguish between venomous snakes and pythons but panics at the sight of anything smooth and coiling. He is no longer responding to the actual threat of danger but to his fear of becoming panicky. Of course, a person who fears a panic state will automatically start to feel panicky, which causes him to become more frightened until he is in a genuinely panic. The self-regulating cycle of the fear reaction has entered a self-sustaining phase where the reaction intensifies itself regardless of the actual threat from the environment.

This account of phobic states needs qualification. With repeated exposure to a threat, most fear responses do fade away but some don't. The aberrant ones intensify until they control the person's life. To be convincing, this model has to show why some people are mortally afraid of frogs whereas most people aren't. Behaviorists would say the person must have had a very bad experience with frogs but this isn't true in the vast majority of cases. I submit that the innate cognitive system has a lot to do with the transition from normal fear response to phobia. Also, the person's physical health at the time of first exposure is important: fears are readily acquired when a person is ill, especially recovering from a debilitating illness such as hepatitis, malaria or dysentery. Finally, there is the factor that some people are simply scared of being anxious, just because they don't know how to control it or where it will end. They become frightened of being frightened, whereas most people know that fears will always fade away. My uncontrolled experiments show that these people often have trouble calming a frightened child or animal as they panic over being frightened themselves.

A panic state is the same reaction as a phobic state, but without the external stimulus. The individual panics over his perception that he is becoming panicky. Being scared is the ultimate threat, just because he knows it will fly out of control and he will be tortured by the worst feelings imaginable. A true panic state simply intensifies until the person is utterly exhausted and it wears itself out. This differs from the phobic states where the individual has a degree of control over how he feels: avoid frogs. By avoidance, the phobic states are kept in a degree of stable instability; in a panic states, however, there is no escape and the terrifying feelings build up and up until the person can barely walk or talk. It is the mental equivalent of a jet engine shaking itself to bits when its control mechanisms are overwhelmed, except that, in panic states, the control mechanisms just are the destructive factor. The person becomes locked in a self-reinforcing state of terror. There is no suggestion whatsoever of a biological defect in his brain. His brain is working fine; it is intensifying his panic nicely, just as it is supposed to do when it perceives a threat. However, the generic response to threats has become the threat itself.

11-4 (c) Paranoid states

The paranoid stance is definitely self-protective, but it hovers uneasily on the borderland between self-help and self-destruction. To an extent, we have to expect danger in daily life, otherwise we would soon be gravy. However, there is a difference between the cognitive sets: "They might be out to get me," versus "They are definitely out to get me." The first injunction merely keeps the individual on his toes while the second leads to a self-reinforcing state of disorder. There is no single rule which, in itself, constitutes the paranoid stance; rather, each person has a unique cluster of views, rules or injunctions which act to protect him in a potentially hostile environment. A cheerful, open person who has never had anything go wrong in life might have only a few rules controlling his level of trust, while a person who has been mistreated will be much more suspicious and defensive. What the paranoid person does not realize is that his behavior influences the environment, inducing the hostility that he didn't want in the first place. That is, a highly defensive posture causes other people to become wary and defensive themselves. Unfortunately, the paranoid man takes this as evidence that his first assessment was right, and he should therefore become more, not less wary. So it intensifies, until he is absolutely convinced everybody is out to get him and, worse still, he has a pile of evidence that is (mostly) true.

There are five mental states which are traditionally taken as variants on the paranoid theme, but practically all of them have a basis in the innate cognitive system. It is for this reason that paranoid disorders are universal. There is not and never will be a single gene (or even a cluster of genes) which controls the level of paranoid thinking. The paranoid or defensive stance ("Only the paranoid survive") is part of the human heritage. How, then, can it be transmitted from one generation to the next? My proposal is this: indirectly. I cannot offer a suggestion as to how a person could have a direct genetic disposition to worrying about police cars slowing down when they pass his house. The cognitive systems involved in making that assessment are so complex that they probably don't even reside on the same chromosomes. However, there is one genetically-influenced factor which could be the mediating factor in all of the paranoid stances: the sense of danger. As a part of the innate cognitive system, the perception of threats is under strong genetic control.

We know that certain animals are more prone to anxiety reactions than others. This is true of breeds of dogs and horses, of different sorts of monkeys, fish, birds and so on. They startle more easily than other breeds or species, meaning the normal distribution of anxiety reactions in these breeds is shifted to the right. It does not suggest that all members of the breed will always be more anxious than all members of the next breed but says there is considerable overlap, just as there is in any genetically-influenced parameter in humans, such as height, intelligence or eye color. The point about the paranoid reactions is that they are crude and biased toward safety, just like the innate response to any perceived threat. The person makes the assessment he is in some sort of danger and then looks around for the evidence. A placid person will soon decide there was no cause for alarm, whereas the anxious person will keep scanning the environment to find evidence to calm himself. But there isn't any. That's what threat responses are about: saving the bacon. The placid person will be less likely to find a hidden threat than the congenitally suspicious. The person who remains on guard, reluctant to settle back again until he is entirely sure, won't sleep very well but he is more likely to survive. However, each time he sees something that might be evidence of danger, his arousal level rises—and rises. Gradually, he shifts into a state of permanent wariness, constantly scanning the environment for threats but unable to accept that there are none. Despite his appearance, the paranoid person is never calm: placid means not on guard, and not on guard means "They could sneak up."

I suggest vigilant anxiety is the core of the paranoid stance. It keeps the person alert to threats but, unfortunately, it produces the evidence that convinces him he needs to become more and more alert and mistrustful. It is a clear example of how the self-regulating cognitive functions can move from being self-protecting to self-destructive. That is, mental pathology does not depend on traumatic events or biochemical defects but results from a small slip in normal mental function. There is a strong element of chance in these types of disorders. Different people (meaning with different genetic make-ups) will react differently to different events. Given a widespread traumatic event, some people will confront it with assurance while others will become increasingly anxious, just because that is their particular constitution (i.e. combination of genetic and experiential factors, both physical and psychological).

Traditionally, psychiatry recognizes five variants of the paranoid stance. They are closely related and it would be very rare to find an individual with just one of the clinical features. The first is the well-known exaggerated sense of persecution and hostility directed at the individual from the environment. This ranges from a slight wariness which really doesn't differ from normality, to full-blown beliefs of persecution. Two warnings are necessary. First, there is no firm demarcation point separating normality from abnormality. Normal depends on time, place, age, culture, etc. Secondly, the person may in fact be persecuted. Does that make him a paranoid nut? This can lead to huge difficulties in dealing with people from different cultures, especially if they have survived wars or other devastation. In addition, there are paranoid cultures in which people see persecution where others would see random events or innocent fun. A particular case is where people interpret another person's mistakes as deliberate attempts at persecution. I often say to my patients: "Don't interpret their incompetence as malice. It's not. They are more likely to be lazy, stupid or ignorant than nasty." This is very important where distressed people have to deal with governments and large corporations.

The second variant is everybody's favorite, conspiracies. Humans, I have said, are pattern detectors *par excellence*. As they say, once is happenstance, twice is coincidence but three times is deliberate. The person who can detect the pattern of danger first will survive, the rest will die. The true conspiracy theorist does not believe in random events: there is no such thing as chance. Everything has a cause, just because everything is potentially dangerous. A committed conspiracy theorist reverses the burden of proof: he doesn't ask for positive proof that two people have conspired against him, he asks for the absolute security of proof that they didn't. The role of anxiety in the paranoid stance is very clear. There is another type of conspiracy theorist which might cause difficulties clinically, the perverse conspiratorialist. Some people don't believe the public explanations for anything, they make a hobby out of trying to prove that something didn't happen the way the authorities say it did. It is as though they want to be the first to "discover the truth" because, very often, they are rather insignificant little people who are misfits of one sort or another. They actually enjoy it, it becomes a game although, like most games, it can become very serious when egos are involved. So, the official explanation of the Kennedy assassination was dismissed as a cover-up; there is that hardy perennial, the belief that the oil majors have bought a patent that allows cars to run on water and are suppressing it; every infection is the result of CIA/KGB/MI5 etc. germ warfare experiments gone wrong (surely these people realize we are on the receiving end of germ warfare all day, every day, but it's the germs that are doing it); don't forget the Protocols of the Elders of Zion, the Shroud of Turin, Nostradamus, UFOs, alien abduction and the rest of this endless genre.

A small but important group are the diet faddists. It is an enduring belief that there is something we can add to or subtract from the diet that will cure anything and everything. The more persistent and more benign the disorder, the more the faddists are certain they can cure it. Left to themselves, these people are harmless but they are rarely content to live on their own concoctions, they have to convert others (and I use the term 'convert' advisedly). They have a special significance for psychiatry, as so many of our conditions are poorly defined, disabling to the sufferers and irksome to the medical people. People will never stop believing that depression can be cured by vitamins or schizophrenia by selenium; that children must avoid red cordial or sugars or natural salicylates; that shark cartilage cures this or chelating agents cure that. Anybody who has listened to an angry mother at a school meeting demanding that the school tuck shop stop stocking white bread or margarine or red ice sweets will realize that this is no ordinary "concerned parent." This is unreasoning fury combined with unyielding self-righteousness, central elements in the paranoid personality. A conspiracy implies secret knowledge, and the paranoid personality believes he or she has it but wicked people are conspiring to conceal it.

This would be funny if it didn't blur across into the dangerously deranged. The Ku Klux Klan genuinely believes that black people are genetically inferior and are out to mix the races (as though whites wouldn't do such things). The former president of South Africa believed (if we know what he believed) that AIDS was a conspiracy by whites to demean blacks, and half a million of his citizens died as a result. Russians were so convinced that the world was trying to take over their country that they had to build a fence to keep their citizens in.

The third big category of paranoid ideas is centered on pathological jealousy. Again, this spreads imperceptibly from the mildest concern about why one's partner spent so long on the phone, to delusional homicidal fury. Pathological jealousy is one of the most dangerous psychiatric disorders of all. It appears to be based in several differing classes of beliefs. One cluster of jealous ideas centers on the idea that the partner cannot be trusted because all members of that sex are promiscuous by nature. That is a simple belief based usually in experience although it may be experience of the wrong sort: if a man has discovered that he can seduce any woman he likes, then he is most unlikely to trust women (this is equally true of women). However, as the Freudians would say, it is a projection: he is attributing to the women the very trait that he displays himself. Beliefs of promiscuity alone can be a problem but, when combined with personal insecurity, it becomes very unstable. A person who believes he is not good enough to keep a partner faithful will be constantly on guard to make sure nobody tries to steal her away. If he also believes that women can't help themselves, then the scene is set for deadly Shakespearian storms.

What has this to do with a cognitive psychology? A lot. In the first place, the paranoid stance just is a belief system. It is a way of classing events in the world, a means of sorting people and things into trustworthy or unreliable, or actually dangerous. A machine can do this but if it classed too many people as untrustworthy, we would not consider it dangerous, only stupid. A simple sorting problem becomes dangerous when it activates emotions, and this is exactly what happens because the sorting process is performed at a crude, intuitive level, namely, the innate cognitive system. Fear of abandonment is a primitive human fear, also seen in all other primates. The need to possess or be possessed by a mate is a powerful drive in practically all species. In humans, it is combined with the hierarchical drive, especially in males: a man without a partner is only half a man, he knows it, everybody knows it, and it hurts. The paranoid stance therefore ranges from a mild, personal quirk right across the emotional spectrum to some of the most basic human drives.

Fourthly, a syndrome of pathological involvement in matters of right and wrong and of justice has long been accepted as a variant paranoid state. I have previously suggested that the concept of fairness is deep-seated in the innate cognitive system, probably via the territorial drive. It can, however, become an obsessive drive to the point where the individual is consumed by the thirst for justice. In fact, it would not be unfair to say these people have only one desire, to crush their opponents, and the law will do nicely, thank you. Again, there is a huge range from a mild, hair-splitting preoccupation with right and wrong, across the spectrum to the vexatious litigant, via the passionate crusader, the inveterate rescuer and the compulsive martyr. This variant depends on the concept of a rule-based human society. If there are no rules, then there is no concept of right or wrong.

However, underlying all the crusaders, litigants, revolutionaries, martyrs and so on is the primitive human belief: "I am right, you are wrong and you must submit to me." This is part of the hierarchical drive, as displayed by chimps and baboons, but humans can tag it to the concept of the rule-based society so that the rulebook becomes a handy weapon. The core of this legalistic variant of the paranoid stance is a burning self-righteousness. The true litigation-minded paranoid sees the law and himself as one and the same thing, which is why they behave so badly when they finally get power. The corollary of "I am right" is "I can do no wrong, so if you oppose me, you must be malicious, and I will destroy you." It also explains why so many of them behave so badly when they think nobody is watching. Martin Luther, who believed so strongly in his vision of right and wrong that he took on the might of the Universal Church, was unusual in that he was apparently faithful to his wife and kept his fingers out of the collection box. Every revolutionary has to be more than a little paranoid, otherwise he would give up and go fishing.

Finally, there is the group which can cause the psychiatrist to want to go fishing, the supernaturalists. A consuming involvement in matters of the supernatural does not include the ordinary church-, mosque- or temple-goers, who believe what they are told and are satisfied with that. However, in every congregation, there is likely to be one member who pores over the texts and claims to have discovered hidden meanings, which sets him at odds with the orthodoxy. Of course, many religious splinter groups are built on the idea of exclusive knowledge of arcane matters, very often under the overwhelming influence of a particularly dominant personality who is venerated as a gifted leader, if not a prophet. Clinically, "prophets" are indistinguishable from those who are not members of a specific group but are convinced they are in touch with the supernatural world. These include the various spiritualists, ghost hunters, crystal gazers, Kirlian photographers and other cranks such as flat-Earthers and colonic irrigators.

People who are intrigued by the supernatural are eccentric, meaning not satisfied with the conventional explanations, and seek their own. That's good, it is the basis of science, but their interest goes far beyond that of a scientist investigating, say, microwave radiation from the Big Bang or a new species of ants that lives only in the stems of certain desert grasses. Where they take leave of boring reality is that they do not accept any limits to their field of study, to their methodology or technology and nor do they accept criticism. In Stevenson's terms [6], they function in a closed intellectual system. They do not allow any evidence to count against their theories, believing to the end that counterevidence can be explained away by the theory; and they respond to criticism by analyzing the critic's motives in terms of their theory. Their conviction that they are right and everybody else is wrong is the same as motivates a great scientist such as Copernicus or Lister, but that is where the parallel ends. Their views are continuous with the milder forms of odd or quirky belief, which are themselves continuous with the frankly deluded. That is, there is no demarcation point between sense and nonsense. It is what they believe and want to investigate. It is normal human curiosity which, I have argued, is part of the innate cognitive system, mated perversely to a passionate self-righteousness and a need to prove everybody else wrong. In fact, that sounds like Newton himself.

There is almost never a pure paranoid type. A vexatious litigant is almost always convinced his enemies are conspiring with the authorities to cheat him of his rights; the jealous man fears that his partner has put a drug in his food to make him impotent; the religious fanatic fears that homosexuals are trying to infiltrate his group; the conspiracy theorist eagerly believes that aliens in UFOs are abducting people for sexual abuse, and so on.

But at the center of the paranoid state is fear: fear of abandonment, of loss of dominance, of being wrong and humiliated. These are primitive fears, mediated by the innate cognitive system. In this respect, the paranoid stance is part of our normal primate heritage, part of our evolutionary survival apparatus but it can go wrong. The normal mechanisms of mental homeostasis may become self-reinforcing, such that the person slips into an increasingly disordered state. Paranoid is, of course, an adjective. It says only that this is the flavor of a person's belief system. Paranoid ideas are very common in personality disorders and in a variety of other conditions. A person can have a paranoid personality, or develop paranoid ideas while depressed, or his self-reinforcing ideas can congeal into true paranoid delusions. Central to this is the idea that we are all paranoid, it is a normal way of thinking that keeps us alive and, without any underlying brain disorder, it can get out of control.

11-5. Conclusion

Years ago, a very prominent British psychiatrist said grumpily: "I don't know how anybody can imagine that the devastation of schizophrenia could be produced by psychological means." However, the old chap didn't have the advantage of living with a desktop computer that regularly tied itself in knots. For us, the idea that a programming fault can halt the most powerful machines in the world is close to second nature: remember the Y2K bug? A simple matter of a missing zero on the date threatened to throw the world into chaos. Similarly, the current economic mess is not the result of a single crop failure or a factory explosion anywhere in the world. Every acre tilled in 2006 is still under cultivation, earthquakes have not devastated the industrial heartlands of the world, nor do famines and plagues stalk the face of the earth, yet the vast and vastly complex international financial system nearly crashed in October 2008. Was it a failure of the world's physical resources, or a programming fault?

I think the problem for the elderly psychiatrist was that he didn't have the first clue of the complexity of human mental life. He still thought in traditional terms, of a little wraith poking its elfin fingers in the cerebral porridge. He could understand the notion of a brain as the central exchange for signals, as he had studied physiology when he was a student in the 1930s. He knew all about galvanic stimulation of pithed toads, and he knew that something had to start the process of movement but he had no idea where or what it was. Looking at a pallid brain gave no indication of what that something might be. Peering at neurons under a microscope was interesting, but where was the energizing soul? How could the richness of daily sensory experience arise from these tiny squiggles? He couldn't imagine it, but he made the classic mistake Schopenhauer saw in his colleagues: "They mistake the limits of their own field of vision for the limits of the world."

There have been many historical examples of people declaring that something was impossible, but the problem lay in their failure of imagination. We don't know how the Greeks took to Archimedes' claim "Give me a fulcrum and I will move the world," but look at it from the point of view his neighbor in the colony of Syracuse. Here we have the world, a vast, flat and immeasurably ponderous creation, around which circle the sun, the moon and the stars, yet this crazy man, who is not averse to running naked through the streets, believes he can move it? Really, what next? Move ahead nearly 2,000 years, and by the simple expedient of sailing due west, Columbus showed that everything the ancients had said about geography was wrong. Closer to home, Ignaz Semmelweiss dared to challenge the establishment with his outrageous claim that they were murdering their patients by infecting them with puerperal fever—and he died for his troubles.

Not so long after, the great Lord Kelvin determined that Darwin's theory of evolution could not possibly be true because the sun would have burned out in the time span Darwin needed to account for speciation. However, he assumed that the sun was made of coal as he had no idea of nuclear energy. Lord Rutherford, who showed where Kelvin erred, damned the industry his research had pioneered just three months before it was shown to be technically feasible: "The energy produced by breaking down the atom," he opined, "is a very poor kind of thing. Anyone who expects a source of power from the transformations of these atoms is talking moonshine." The Nobel laureate immunologist, Sir Macfarlane Burnett, showed equal aptitude in gloomy forecasts. In 1949, he announced: "I can see no hope at present of such a vaccine being produced... I have adopted a frankly defeatist attitude towards the problem of poliomyelitis... No means of controlling poliomyelitis is at present visible." He was similarly glum for the prospects of one of the modern growth industries: "I can see no practical application of molecular biology to human affairs... DNA is a tangled mass of linear molecules in which the informational content is quite inaccessible."

Failures of imagination go both ways, of course, the most spectacular crashes being in politics and finance. Wars and depressions do not just happen. They are started by people who fail to foresee where their clever plans might run into difficulties. Did the architects of the invasion of Iraq really submit their ideas to critical evaluation? Did the nameless people who invented complex financial derivatives such as CDOs and CDSs ask themselves what would happen if people lost confidence in them? The actuaries in Lehmann Bros believed the chances of a breakdown in their risk management lay further than 25 standard deviations from the mean. Did they never suspect their calculations were wrong, that humans can't actually measure anything that far from the mean? Human inventions, even mathematics, can go wrong in unsuspected ways.

What is the point of these historical rebukes? The point is that science has a habit of leap-frogging obstructions. A person who has worked successfully in the area for many years hits an intellectual block. His training and experience does not allow him to see a way around it. That is what the word "block" means: unable to move ahead. Instead of thinking there may be some shortcoming in his approach, because that would necessitate abandoning some precious beliefs, he announces the end of the line. However, another person, often a neophyte, who doesn't have the same emotional commitment to the old methods, comes along, has a quick look at it and says brightly: "But why don't we go this way instead?" The newcomer sees an conceptual bridge joining the observations where everybody else sees despair. Predictably, the old guard are never quite as grateful as they could be.

Psychiatry is not immune to naysayers: "I don't know how anybody can imagine that the devastation of schizophrenia could be produced by psychological means." That is simply a failure of imagination, mistaking his own intellectual limitations for a general rule of the universe because we now have a concept bridging the gap between the brain and psychosis. It doesn't come from medicine. In another field, we have moved a long way since this claim, a very, very long way. An entire new realm of discourse has opened, one in which the previously sacrosanct processes of human intellect are increasingly handled by machines. Machines are now our drudges, leaving us, as Turing hoped, to fix our minds on higher things although we will never know if he had internet pornography in mind. However, we can be certain that psychiatrists of the older generation, who were determined to purge psychiatry of psychoanalytic pseudoscience, did not understand the growing power of machine-based intelligence.

Thirty years ago, when the DSM-III committees met to decide the direction of the new psychiatry, they knew that if they wished to avoid the trap of unrestrained psychologizing, they had to avoid any hint of mentalism. As their guarantee, they proposed a rigid biological reductionism which could not, they were sure, be taken over by armchair philosophers. Now, having lived through three decades of fervent biologism, its limits are coming into clearer focus. With the advantage of watching Moore's Law (that computing power doubles every eighteen months) in action, we know that fantastic computing power can be compressed into tiny machines. We don't have any problem with the idea of machines making decisions on increasingly complex matters. As long as the problem can be defined in terms of yes/no questions, a machine can handle it. We are fully familiar with the notion of connecting banks of machines to produce much larger computing entities, such as the internet. We use today's machines to produce even more powerful ones for tomorrow, so that the total power of human effort is now increasing exponentially. We also never question that any machines we can make will eventually break down. With very complex systems such as the internet, the idea of problems amplifying themselves, until the system crashes to an ignoble halt, is now yesterday's news. The data-processing capacity of the brain is one such "very complex system." There is no innate reason why it, too, should not "crash to a halt."

Throughout this work, I have made no secret of the fact that the biocognitive model does not have an answer to the question of sensory experience. To fill the gap, I have suggested that conscious experience arises by a complex manipulation of sensory input by a powerful virtual algorithm generated by the brain's huge data processing capacity. I doubt whether we could ever know the ultimate cause of the realm of experience, just because the codes by which it is generated may be beyond our reach. That is an open question, but it doesn't affect the main thrust of this work, which is to show how the rapid, silent manipulation of information by the brain produces the decisions we need to survive. There is nothing magical about these processes yet, like any other mechanized process, neuronal decisions can go wrong. This is where the failure of imagination becomes a brake on scientific understanding of mental disorder. If we believe that the crucial decisions which initiate behavior come from a soul, then there is no way that soul can be wrong, so mental disorder has to come from the brain. But if the "soul" can be reduced to a matter of information processing, then we immediately open the door to a non-biological causation of mental disorder.

In this chapter, I have given two examples of how vicious circles produce self-intensifying psychiatric syndromes. In psychiatry, anxiety states are of huge importance, not just because they are so common but also because they are so central to many other syndromes. The DSM-IV approach does not recognize this because it is allegedly a behavioral analysis only, mapping surface syndromes without giving thought to the underlying processes that are generating those syndromes (I say alleged because it is behavioral except when inconvenient, such as the post-traumatic states). From the theoretical point of view, the anxiety states are interesting because the negative feedback loop extends from mind to body, and then back again. This loop can be broken at a number of points, which is of major therapeutic significance.

The paranoid states, on the other hand, remain wholly within the cognitive realm. Conceptually, the word paranoid applies to a totally different class of mental events from emotional terms such as anxiety and depression. Paranoid is an adjective which applies to the way we interpret events, i.e. it constitutes only a cognitive stance on the world, or a way of classifying information, but it has no emotional content itself. Paranoid states are often associated with intense emotion, but the emotions are strictly secondary to the cognitive appraisal of events and are enormously variable. There is no such thing as "paranoia." That is reification, akin to saying that a good person has a lot of goodness in him, or a bad person is full of evil.

Paranoid states are self-reinforcing or amplifying because they influence the person to search the environment for particular events, which he then adds to his sum of life experiences. At the same time, he routinely denies or ignores any evidence likely to contradict his persecutory mental set. Moreover, his views tend to be self-confirming or self-fulfilling because the paranoid individual modifies the behavior of his social environment, further influencing his experiences. Crucially, there is no theoretical limit to the extent to which a person's mental state can be driven in a particular direction by these means. Each adverse incident influences his future perceptions, and each of these influences other mental functions in an unpredictable manner.

I have used different terms for this phenomenon: self-reinforcing, self-amplifying, self-fulfilling, vicious circle, negative feedback loops, and so on, but they are properly classed as recursive functions. This means that a function operates continuously, taking as its starting point the end-point of its last iteration. Thus, a tiny variation can be amplified exponentially until either it reaches a state of stable instability, or it destroys the system. A spectacular physical example occurred in 1940, when a wind blowing at a particular speed over the newly-built Tacoma Narrows Bridge induced an aero-elastic flutter which destroyed the bridge. The physics was quite simple, as the external periodic frequency of the wind matched and amplified the natural structural frequency of the suspension bridge, until it collapsed. The chain reaction of a nuclear explosive is another well-known example, with the Chernobyl disaster a clear illustration of what happens when the controls on a self-sustaining reaction are lifted. Psychologically, stampedes of social animals, including humans at gatherings such as sporting, religious or political meetings, are examples of fear feeding upon fear until the previously disciplined mass of animals explodes in frenzy. There are many examples of self-amplifying excess in financial history, including the Dutch tulip mania of 1636, the British South Sea Bubble of 1720 and the Mississippi Company boom of 1719. The current financial crisis is a classic example of self-reinforcing greed building up and up until it collapsed abruptly.

I propose that the concept of self-reinforcing feedback loops represents the conceptual bridge between observations and thought which allows us to bypass the older psychiatric generation's failure of imagination. Just as the mathematics of levers bypassed the Syracusean skeptics, and solar nuclear energy bypassed Kelvin's skepticism of Darwin's theories, or computing power allowed us to disentangle DNA codes, so too the concept of recursive functions operating in the psychological realm allows us to bridge the conceptual gap between the brain and the devastation of the paranoid psychoses.

There can be no argument with the general notion of recursive functions. The concept applies to any complex data processor. Because of this well-established phenomenon, *nobody can prove that psychological factors cannot produce the furthest reaches of the paranoid states*. So the old British psychiatrist now has to revisit his opinion about the causation of mental disorder, even very severe disorders such as schizophrenia. If the brain processes data, there is no *a priori* reason why the mind cannot arise as the result of cerebral data-processing. But anybody who accepts that the mind is ultimately a matter of data processing cannot deny that self-amplifying errors can (and almost certainly will) arise whenever data are processed. From this point, it is no major conceptual jump to the notion that severe mental disorders can arise purely as a matter of self-reinforcing errors of the processes by which data are manipulated in the brain. The generic name for "self-reinforcing errors of data processing" is *circus vitiosus*: let us shout it from the rooftops because it crashes through the limits of imagination which have confined psychiatry to the Procrustean bed of DSM-IV.

12

The Culture of Complacency

*"The truth will set you free.
But first, it will piss you off."*
*Gloria Steinem**

12-1. Introduction

Does psychiatry have a future? If it continues on its present course, where will it be by the time today's young psychiatrists are ready to retire? On present trends, there won't be many of them left. The number of vacant training posts in psychiatry is rising, the average age of new trainees is rising, and the average age of practicing psychiatrists is rising even faster. It is a graying profession. Nowadays, psychiatry is often a second career, the choice of general practitioners who are tired of the long hours and hope for something quieter, of people changing careers or of women coming back to medicine after having had their families. It is also one of the main routes for foreign graduates to gain restricted registration, as local graduates are rarely interested in working in rural centers. The secular trends are crystal clear: when I entered psychiatry, most new psychiatrists in Australia were young, local, male graduates working full-time. These days, the demographics are that newly-qualified psychiatrists are more likely to be older, more likely to be female, and more likely to be foreign graduates, undertaking second careers,

---

* On legal advice, the original version of this chapter was drastically revised. My advice was that the chapter was suitable for publication in the US, where it would be protected by the freedom of speech amendment, by public interest and by the fact that, in the torrent of anti-medical literature, nobody would notice anyway. However, Britain and Australia are different. Because Australian and British defamation laws are so poorly defined, they serve the purpose of reducing comment on major issues just by intimidating authors. On advice, I therefore elect not to have to spend the next four years defending myself against vexatious litigation. This is purely on the basis that it would be vexatious to me, not because anything I have said on matters of grave public importance is false or wilfully injurious to anybody.

often part-time, and often more interested in academic or administrative advantage than clinical work.

It is striking the numbers of younger psychiatrists who do not undertake full-time clinical work. Increasingly, they work part-time and then work in administrative or supervisory roles which reduces their clinical experience even further. Today's trainees are most likely to be taught and supervised by people who take what can only be described as an unhurried view of the profession. Even as recently as when I trained, teachers were busy people winding down after long and productive careers whereas their modern counterparts have cut the ballyhoo of clinical life and headed straight for the academic/administrative path. This is cause for very great concern: if psychiatry is seen as the path to an easy life as a part-time specialist, where doctors spend more time in meetings with each other than in meeting patients, then its standing in the community will fall—even lower. Granted, it suits the psychologists, nurses, social workers and various others if psychiatrists remove themselves from the arena but it will accelerate our decline to irrelevance. If the teachers teach only what they've read in books, then the students' curiosity will shrivel. I have no doubt that teachers with broad and worldly clinical experience are far more tolerant of intellectual diversity than those without. How, then, will psychiatry attract the bright young graduates (male and female, local and foreign) who will push impatiently at the limits of our knowledge?

Daily, we hear about the epidemic of depression afflicting the Western world, about rising rates of suicide, alcohol and drug addiction, of post-traumatic states and so on, but who is going to treat these looming disasters? More to the point, who is going to be bright enough to find the errors in today's "evidence-based models of problem-oriented, outcome-driven, multidisciplinary team triage interventions cost-effectively meeting the service delivery unit's mission statement and program goals for consumers and key stake-holders"? Who is going to be bold enough to say that this obsession with high-sounding jargon conceals a theoretical black hole? Who is going to stand up in the annual congresses in the luxury resorts and demand of the keynote speaker: "But what is the name of the scientific model of mental disorder your figures and tests address? Show us three seminal references where the model is set out as a series of testable propositions, and show when and where there was a debate in which this model was compared critically with its competitors. And if you can't answer those questions, Professor sir, then your brand of psychiatry has no basis in science."

As a profession, psychiatry has nothing approximating an accepted theory of mental life. For a century and a half, they have been satisfied with little more than collections of shibboleths such as ids and egos, chemical imbalances, conditioned reflexes and biopsychosocial models, all the while managing to convince the fee-paying general public that there was something of substance behind their impenetrable jargon. Can this continue until today's young psychiatrists are checking their pension accounts?

12-2. How Psychiatry Fails To Qualify As Science.

12-2 (a). A cloak of respectability.

Modern psychiatry has the trappings of a successful field of scientific medicine. Just like cardiologists, obstetricians and neurosurgeons, psychiatrists have their own professional bodies, their five year training programs, their degrees and gowns, their citations and awards, their committees and research programs. They have university departments and benevolent foundations, congresses and journals, public relations campaigns, high-level planning meetings with governments and an entire industry devoted to writing the systems of classification that passes for psychiatric thinking. Eric Dean noted: "The history of psychiatry has, in a sense, been the history of various medical men and theoreticians attempting to understand mental pathology by means of rigorous classification" [1, p34]. There is also a second industry devoted to publishing the huge lists of throwaway handbooks of multi-authored, evidence-based community interventions for survivors of sexual abuse by garden gnomes. It would be easy to say that this is all pointless but there is a point: over this frantic activity looms the shadow of the biggest, most powerful lobby of all, the drug industry.

Anybody who has ever been to a psychiatric conference, with its busy buzz of concerned middle-aged, middle-class people will be impressed by the paraphernalia: take away the word psychiatry and replace it with nephrology or pediatrics and there would be no great difference. There are lectures and workshops, research presentations and continuing education points. People hurry from conference hall to seminar room where droning lecturers project page after page of dense statistics on their research. Yet a brief enquiry would reveal that two vital things are missing: a formal scientific theory or model that gives the paraphernalia a goal, and the searing blowtorch of criticism to make the intellectually-complacent jerk awake. Without these two things, the whole panoply of science is a charade. This is why Dean could conclude that curiosity in psychiatry has been replaced by an industry of classification. I believe this to be the truth of modern psychiatry but it is a truth that really pisses psychiatrists off. It makes them very angry—but never so angry that they will settle the matter once and for all by naming their theory of mental disorder and giving its critics a free lecture theater.

12-2 (b). "Trust me, I'm a doctor."

Modern psychiatry is a hollow charade. These are very strong words but, because of the overwhelming importance of psychiatry in the community, it is the inescapable duty of anybody who believes there may be faults to say so openly. We can start with the extreme case:

> Fraud: *noun* 1. Deliberate deception, trickery, or cheating intended to gain an advantage. 2. An act or instance of such deception. 3.Something false or spurious: *his explanation was a fraud.*

This seems reasonably clear: fraud is a deliberate attempt by somebody who knows the truth to lead another person into believing something other than the truth, for the purpose of gaining some sort of benefit. Does modern psychiatry meet this definition? Strictly speaking, it does not. The definition depends on two people, two mental states and an unjustified or improper benefit for one. Person A has belief state Q_A which happens to be the truth. With careful planning, A attempts to induce in person B a separate belief state Q_B (which is not Q_A) because, as long as B believes Q_B, then A can gain a benefit or advantage for himself.

If we try to apply this definition to the state of modern psychiatry, we run into a problem. With regard to mental disorder, psychiatrist Dr. A believes proposition Q_A: Mental disorder is a product of brain disorder such that a specific brain disorder is both necessary and sufficient for a particular mental disorder. Dr. A accepts this as true without reservation. He therefore attempts to induce in his patient, Ms. B, a like belief state which, if she accepts it, will result in A getting an advantage, mostly money and prestige. However, B's new belief state Q_B does not differ from A's belief state Q_A. In fact, A's advantage lies in convincing B to accept Q_A wholeheartedly, not to conceal it from her. Dr. A must convince Ms. B to accept what he believes, otherwise she will go to see somebody else. Thus, if anybody were to say that modern psychiatry is a fraud, the charge probably wouldn't stick.

However, there is more to this question than Dr. A's beliefs about mental disorder. Assume that Ms. B is in dire mental straits from misery and wants somebody to help her. She is sent to psychiatrist Dr. A who announces: "I am an expert in your kind of dire straits. Upon my wall is a large certificate which pronounces me an expert so, for a consideration, I shall heal you." From his reading of the psychiatric journals and from attending conferences, Dr. A believes that misery is a genuine disease state caused by an unseen chemical imbalance of the brain. He does not question this truth. He is highly desirous of Ms. B believing him otherwise she will not accept treatment, the effect being that she remains unhappy and A will not get paid. So he attempts to induce in Ms. B a belief state Q_B that is a facsimile of his own belief state Q_A. Of course, the good doctor can't actually see or test for the chemical imbalance in Ms. B's brain but all his books and journals and all his colleagues agree it is there so he is happy with that. Because Ms. B isn't really in a position to argue (there's that certificate, after all), she takes the tablets and pays Dr. A, who doesn't doubt that what he has told her is true. So where is the wrongdoing? It all hinges on A's claim that he is not just an ordinary person, he is an *expert*.

The psychiatrist could have said to his patient: "My dear lady, misery is a perfect bore, you have my full sympathy. However, despite the many bravura certificates on my wall, misery remains a mystery. I do not have a theory of what causes it. However, I do know that 61% of people who take this particular medicament will eventually stop moping and get back to work. And if this one doesn't work, we'll just go through the pharmacy until we find something that seems to do the trick."

Now if the good Dr. A said that, which is a rough approximation of the truth in psychiatry, Ms. B might not be sufficiently impressed to hand over some of her hard-earned dollars and might even spread it around town that A doesn't know what he is talking about. Would the lady be justified in spreading this rumor? She may be, because part of the definition of expert is "knows what he is talking about," thus:

> Expert: *noun.* 1. A person who has extensive skill or knowledge in a particular field...

Certificates do not confer knowledge, they merely advertise it. Extensive skill or knowledge in the field of mental disorder is what makes a psychiatrist an expert, and allows him to charge accordingly. When a psychiatrist says to a patient: "Your unhappy state is caused by a chemical imbalance of the brain," he is not just saying something he believes to be true that week, or something he hopes the patient will be silly enough to believe (and pay for). He is also saying: "I am an expert because I have studied all aspects of this field. What I say is right and anybody who contradicts me is wrong. If you think your misery is caused by having buck teeth as a child or could be cured by talking, you too are wrong. Take these and come back in a month."

An expert doesn't just diagnose what is wrong with the patient, he goes much further. He says: "This is the truth of what is wrong with you. It is not anything else because not only do I know the truth, I also know what is false and I can tell the difference between truth and falsity. Through my superior knowledge, you will gain a benefit and not a disadvantage." It is at this point that modern psychiatry disqualifies itself as science because modern psychiatrists do not know "all that is true and all that is false" about mental disorder. They know only what they believe to be true: the rest, they dismiss as unimportant. That is, when Dr. A says to the sorrowful Ms. B: "You have a chemical imbalance of the brain," he is also implying to her: "...and it is not your suppressed grievance against your mother, nor is your husband's jealousy a factor, nor are you a mess of conflicting beliefs and ambitions from your dysfunctional family background. Tablets, and only tablets, will cure you." It is at this point that psychiatrists stop being experts because psychiatry does not have a theory which allows its practitioners to say anything like this, and their training has not equipped them to question the prevailing biological model.

Next question: As experts on mental disorder, should psychiatrists know that they don't have a general theory of mental disorder? Of course they should. That is what the word expert means. So why don't they know that discomforting fact? Unfortunately, this question moves from my field to the field of social psychology. It becomes a question of the sociology of closed societies, why a group of otherwise sensible and well-educated people should believe one proposition to be exclusively true when they haven't canvassed the options. Not only has orthodox psychiatry not explored all the options but it dismisses them from the outset. They are like the brilliant Lord Kelvin, who dismissed the theory of evolution as a load of rubbish because it conflicted with his deeply-held views on the nature of the universe. His mind was closed to the possibility that there was more to the universe than his long and productive life had taught him, yet he was soon shown to be wrong (apparently, Kelvin really did believe the sun was made of coal; he knew its diameter, so why didn't he work out how much oxygen it would need to burn before he upbraided Darwin?).

This is why psychiatrists should be very careful about claiming that all mental disease is brain disease: there may be alternatives but the vast majority of modern psychiatrists will never know because they believe the question is closed. It is one thing for a closed group to agree with each other that the sun is made of coal or that all mental disorder is brain disorder *and that no other explanation is possible*; it is something else again to convince the general public to believe it as well. It is at that point that the conduct of the modern institution of psychiatry takes leave of normal scientific ethics. It is improper to claim to be an expert without doing what experts must do to qualify as experts: look critically at *all* the evidence. This is a dangerous point for psychiatry because, if it were willful, it would amount to fraud. I think it is just group stupidity, a bit of arrogance mixed with intellectual sloth and a puerile fear of saying "In all honesty, we don't really know, our theories aren't good enough."

I suggest this peculiar position has arisen because psychiatry is part of allopathic medicine yet its subject matter is removed from the field of mainstream medicine. That is, psychiatrists train as physicians using the tried and proven theories and methods of reductionist science, but then jump to a field (mental life) which has never been shown to be amenable to a reductionist analysis. Biological psychiatry, of course, is the most overt attempt to force the subject matter of psychiatry into the reductionist framework but my case is that it has failed, and failure was inevitable. Unfortunately, the people who have taken control the profession are not open to persuasion that there might be something wrong with their approach and methods, and the forms of training they have devised. Without any attempt at critical analysis, without any discussion, they are satisfied that the general and specific approaches which are successful in, say, orthopedics, can be lifted *holus bolus* into the conceptually different field of mental life, without restriction and with no more risk of failure than in orthopedics. Moreover, they are bitterly antagonistic to any suggestions that there may be some logical weaknesses in their approach to the problem of mental disorder. In fact, they are just as antagonistic as the psychoanalysts and behaviorists were to challenges to their self-appointed intellectual supremacy. I believe it is wrong to claim to be an expert without bothering to conduct oneself like an expert, meaning carefully examining both sides of the argument and arriving at a balanced decision on vexed or complex questions. People who take a strong stance without looking at the options are not experts, they are ideologues, thus:

> Ideologue: *noun* ... 3. (philos) a person who believes an idea or set of ideas that is false, misleading or held for the wrong reasons but is believed with such conviction as to be irrefutable.

Many members of the general public would be greatly aggrieved if, having paid for science, they realized they had been handed ideology. They might start to question whether their hard-earned taxes should continue to subsidize such a profession in future.

12-2 (c). "Against dogma disguised as science, objectivity fails." [2, p98]

The question then arises: how is this bizarre state of affairs maintained? We have to start somewhere, and I see the following list as certain points in an uncertain firmament:

1. The question of the causation of mental disorder is conceptually very complex;

2. A formal proof of the causation of mental disorder waits upon a convincing theory of mind;

3. We do not yet have a convincing theory of mind;

4. Therefore the question of the causation of mental disorder remains open;

5. It is ethically highly improper to state or imply that the question of the causation of mental disorder is settled;

6. By a variety of means, orthodox psychiatry states and implies that the question of the causation of mental disorder is settled.

Biological psychiatrists might object to point (1): "There is nothing complex about it at all," they would reply. "Mental disorder reduces directly to brain disorder." That, however, is an ideological assumption, so we can overlook that objection and move to a potentially more serious charge.

The potential weak point in this argument is point (2). A committed biological psychiatrist might argue that it is an empirical fact that, for each particular mental disorder, there is an underlying biological defect in the brain which should be discovered before long. However, something that hasn't yet been discovered is not yet an empirical fact; it remains a heart-felt ambition, and yearning won't convert it into reality. Moreover, that argument depends entirely on the truth of the categorical system of mental disorder: if, as a matter of fact, there are no true categories of mental disorder, then the biological case fails. That is, if mental disorder does not consist of separate categories (schizophrenia and the affective psychoses, say, are simply different ways of presenting the same underlying condition; the personality disorders are dimensionally distributed and so on), then there can't be a one-to-one relationship between supposed biochemical lesions and the clinical pictures of mental disorder. I have previously argued that the case for a categorical distribution of mental disorders is simply wrong, and there is no lack of support for this view. So the one chance for a biological psychiatrist to negate the points above lacks any convincing support.

We can take this further. Assume for a moment that the categorical model of mental disorder has finally gone the way of the psychoanalytic formulations in the old DSM-II. In its place, the new orthodoxy is that mental disorders consist of the extremes of a multifactorial range of normality, in the same way as *body habitus* consists of a huge, multifactorial range of normality. Each of what were once seen as separate disorders blurs across its neighbors, with no demarcation point between normality and abnormality. Under these circumstances, could there ever be a strictly biochemical or genetic cause for mental disorder? In a sense, there could, but it isn't what people expect. By definition, the genes for mental disorder would not be distinct from the genes for mental order, they would vary continuously. That is, the genes of mental disorder cannot be separated from those of the normal mind, i.e. the genes for mental disorder would be the same genes as for the mind; but since there are no genes for mind, that would mean the genes for brain. Therefore, the genes for mental disorder would be none other than the genes for the normal brain.

Specifically, this means mental disorder arises from the normal brain only by way of disturbances of the normal mind, i.e. mental disorder is just that: psychologically-determined disorder of the mind, not disorder of the brain *per se*. This closes another avenue for the biological model of mental disorder, thereby strengthening point (2).

Therefore, we arrive at:

7. Ethically, orthodox psychiatry is acting in a highly improper manner.

This is hardly a novel claim but, to test this point, let us revisit a major plank to psychiatry's claim to scientific status, its publishing industry. I have said (Chap. 3) that one of the major functions of the psychiatric publishing industry is epistemological, i.e. it is the means by which error is discovered and eliminated. From that particular function flows scientific progress. However, if there is no agreed scientific model of mental disorder, then there can be no error. If you send me to the shop to buy something, and I buy oranges, you cannot claim I have erred. But declaring a model is only half of the epistemological function of publication. We set up a model, and then we attack it. Criticism, as I have said, is the very engine of scientific progress: no criticism, no progress. This is why psychiatry is stalled in an intellectual siding: it has uncoupled its engine. The important question here is: Where do we find the engine? It should be institutionalized in the psychiatric publishing industry but, as I have shown [3], that particular branch of the psychiatric establishment doesn't see any need for criticism. As far as the majority of editorial boards are concerned, they are just a little short of the final mopping up phase in the war against mental disorder. They have the tools, they have the people and they have the map; all they have to do is follow the path to a golden, chemical future. They are completely wrong.

Unjustified and unjustifiable claims by people such as Eric Kandel (see Chap. 1), that biology will tell us all we need to know about humans, put psychiatry in the same position as physics in 1886. At that time, mainstream physicists believed that they had solved most of the major problems of the universe and there was just a bit of mopping up to do. However, in 1887, a famous negative experiment by two researchers in the US, Albert Michelson and Edward Morley, showed that there could not be a luminiferous ether as the basis for propagation of light. This eventually led to a total reappraisal of the nature of the universe, sometimes called the Second Scientific Revolution. In the same vein, today's biological psychiatrists are very comfortable with the idea that they are closing on a complete understanding of human affairs by means of a complete understanding of the human brain. The idea behind reductionist biologism is that, if we know everything there is about the brain, then we will *ipso facto* know everything there is to know about the mind, including disorders of the mind.

This is where the problem of criticism arises, because most of the editors of the majority of mainstream journals in psychiatry are not appointed on the basis of their hostility to the prevailing paradigm. As it is presently structured, the inevitable outcome of the psychiatric publishing industry is such as to filter criticism, leaving only a stream of bland and non-contentious biological and statistical papers addressing an undeclared model. How come nobody notices this is the very antithesis of the critical mode demanded by the scientific ethos? As Chap. 3 shows, it is overwhelmingly obvious that the major journals carefully sidestep the question of what their (very expensive) research is addressing. According to its website, the *British Journal of Psychiatry* has twenty-five editors and assistant editors and forty-six international advisers. It also has immediate access to perhaps hundreds of reviewers. There is no question that all of these highly-educated and highly-paid people would regard themselves as "top echelon." The surprise is that not one of them should raise the question: "But is what we are doing actually science? Let us define science, and see whether our vision of psychiatry meets that definition."

I have suggested that the reason these people feel so comfortable with their performance is actually a question of social psychology, but does that excuse them? These are not just lay-people, nor even run-of-the-mill psychiatrists, they are supposed to be the best the system can bring forth. I won't argue that point; all I will say is that if the best we can manage is a set of people who simply don't know how science is conducted, then we had better scrap the whole deal and start again. In industry and technology, this is known as "basic process re-engineering." It means sitting down with a blank sheet of paper and asking: "What are we trying to do, and what is the best way of going around it?" So, if we want to produce a system where psychiatry progresses, and the only means of ensuring progress is by publication and a intellectual free-for-all, then what would be the best way of going about it? Immediately, it is clear that having a self-selecting clique of people, with no training in the philosophy of science, making major philosophical assumptions (such as Guze's "There cannot be a psychiatry which is too biological") about the nature and direction of the most difficult field of all, is simply a recipe for going nowhere. The purpose of studying theory in psychiatry is to avoid being deceived by psychiatrists (attr. Joan Robinson). With remarkably few exceptions, psychiatrists do not study theory. They grasp it, but they don't know what they are grasping. Given the widespread suspicion that exists about psychiatry, some members of the general public might therefore wonder whether the editorial boards were deliberately attempting to mislead the general public.

I discern a problem of definition here. Deception presupposes that they know better, but I don't believe they do. Once again, they can plead that, since they believe in biological psychiatry, it is not false to broadcast that biological psychiatry will "deliver the goods." The belief licenses the claim. They believe this just as Lord Kelvin believed the sun was made of coal, and other physicists of his time believed in the ether. The belief does not, however, license the active suppression of criticism. I do not believe the editorial boards lock the doors and then agree: "OK, chaps, this is our plan. We only publish stuff supporting the biological model or we're all out of a job." Psychiatrists are not mere conspirators and they are not lacking intelligence. Rather, theirs is the conspiracy of the like-minded, an insipid reluctance to look beyond the obvious for fear it may disturb their shared complacency.

I do, however, believe there is a tacit agreement by many editorial boards that they have a firm grip on the correct model of mental disorder and, on the rare occasion criticism is needed, they are the best people to look after it. This they do by inviting sober, balanced people (read: people like themselves) to handle it in a calm and mature way (unlike their opponents). Since it appears that the members of editorial boards are chosen just because they are the sorts of people who are unlikely to want to pull the whole edifice down, there is a deeper, unspoken meeting of minds to the effect that public squabbling is inappropriate. They see it as ill-mannered and likely to bring the field into disrepute. They appear to have the view that great scientists are all sober, balanced and well-mannered people. Perhaps they are, but only after they have crushed their opponents: "Science has been an arena in which men have striven for two goals: to understand the world, and to achieve recognition for their personal efforts in doing so" [2, p212].

Now the nature of the problem becomes clearer. If anybody were to ask any member of any editorial board of any psychiatric journal of the value of criticism in the advancement of science, that member would surely reply that criticism is very valuable and should be encouraged. If he were then asked: "So what does your journal do to promote criticism?" the member would probably reply: "I'd have to say we don't really see that much. There's broad agreement that modern psychiatry is on the right path."

"But," the interlocutor would continue, "what about those who don't agree? Is there a place for them?"

At this, the editorial chap may venture a smile: "I don't believe it is the role of our journal to cater to a few malcontents," he may say. "You are aware, of course, that some people still oppose the theory of evolution. Does the *Journal of Molecular Genetics* give them space? I don't believe it does, nor do I believe it should. My editorial board and I are in the same position. There is no serious question as to the nature of psychiatry as a science. You can survey all the psychiatric journals. How much criticism of the standard model do you find? Don't you think that says something?"

It certainly does say something, but nothing complimentary to the bulk of the psychiatric publishing industry. It says that by a consistent policy of placing obstacles in the way of criticism, the publishing industry has cultivated a self-perpetuating impression of unanimity. Anyone who challenges the industry is accused of being antagonistic to science. The failure of the various editorial boards to recognize the role of criticism in driving science to better models fosters the notion in readers (and authors, of course) that criticism is not just unnecessary, but is likely to impede progress in understanding mental disorder. The correct model, they say, is in place; attacking it is destructive, and critics should not be allowed to detract from the progress of science. However, it is not possible to claim that criticism is an essential part of science, and then act as though psychiatry does not need criticism. There may be some members of the editorial boards of some establishment journals who believe that the modern statistical-biological approach is wrong but there still remains the unassailable fact of an almost total absence of critical thinking in all mainstream journals. It is at this point that psychiatry takes leave of the field of science and becomes a pretence of science.

12-2 (d) End of the road for Maudsley's dictum.

"Mental disease is brain disease," or so Henry Maudsley announced *ex vacuo* about 150 years ago. He offered no proof of his claim and nobody since has bothered to look too closely at it. For most of the time, the idea of a biological psychiatry was "just there," embraced by the huge mental hospitals but ignored by the intellectuals of university life and of private practice. However, with the collapse of the psychoanalytic tradition and the demise of behaviorism in the 1970s, the field was wide open. Into the void strode the biological reductionists whose simple formula promised progress where the other theories were mired in hair-splitting.

The biological model of psychiatry has reached the end of its road. It promised so much but delivered so little, and all the while it is leading to the intellectual impoverishment of a critically-important specialty. Medical students, trainees and young psychiatrists are slowly coming to see that psychiatry isn't like the other fields of science they have studied. They know that science is important because it is the only way we have of distinguishing a reliable process from chance success but more and more, they are seeing our field as simply wandering in circles. In an editorial in the *Australian and New Zealand Journal of Psychiatry*, the Journal editor, Sydney Bloch [4] opined: "...it is salutary to note in the article on the level of interest in psychiatry among medical students... that an unattractive feature of our profession is its 'perceived absence of a scientific foundation.' This is clearly not an accurate portrayal..." Bloch (who was appointed as editor, not elected) was wrong; the students correctly recognized that scientific truth is not established by dint of repetition of a falsehood. The present conduct of psychiatry is not science because it cannot lead to a viable model of mental disorder: "Now the essence of the scientific spirit is criticism. It tells us that whenever a doctrine claims our assent, we should reply, 'Take it if you can compel it.'" (Thomas Huxley, 1893).

No criticism, no progress. The general public has good reason to feel very angry about that.

12-3. Is There A Future For Psychiatry?

So what does the future hold for psychiatry? I don't know, I'm no better at predicting the future than anybody else. But I do believe that, if we continue on our present course, psychiatry will eventually slide into complete irrelevance. However, if we adopt a new model of mental disorder, one based firmly in the idea that the human mind is a real thing which is not reducible to the brain that generates it, then, at the very least, we have a future. Our teachers were hypnotized by the idea of a mechanistic psychiatry that would answer all the vast problems of mental disorder with a clear, simple formula. It failed. It is now up to the rising generation of psychiatrists to move into theoretical areas, such as self-controlling cognition, which dumbfounded their professors. Revolutions are produced, not by dramatic gesture, but by tediously undermining the foundations of the *status quo*.

The biocognitive model outlined in these pages is far and away the most complex and far-reaching model in the history of psychiatry. It has a breadth and explanatory scope which eclipses anything we have had before. I don't doubt for a moment that it will be found deficient in some, many or even all areas but it represents a huge leap toward the goal of a rational theory of mental disorder. It restores humanity to psychiatry by integrating the biological, psychological and cultural aspects of human life. Granted it is complex, but so are the problems of psychiatry. As Henry Mencken noted: "For every complex problem, there is an answer that is clear, simple, and wrong." Our patients don't need any more "clear, simple" answers to the complex questions of psychiatry.

Epilogue

*"No spell, however potent, can withstand for long the assault of a
skeptical reflection. That is why it is the skeptic and not the believer who
is in the end our savior."*
George Orwell: Homage to Catalonia.

These two books, *Humanizing Madness* and now *Humanizing Psychiatry*,
are the culmination of thirty-five years of struggling with an idea. The idea is
that there has to be an explanation of human distress which avoids the
supernatural yet which preserves our humanity. Every time I tried to tackle
that idea, I was led to questions of philosophy, yet my medical training had
done nothing to prepare me for these types of questions. So I began to drift
further from the mainstream of psychiatry but there was no support, no
interest, no encouragement from the psychiatric establishment in Australia. It
wasn't just Australia: everywhere I looked seemed the same. Psychiatry was
falling under the sway of the American biological model to the extent that
questions of humanity didn't rate a mention. By about 1985, it was very
obvious to me that there was no future in pursuing these ideas. Reluctantly, I
decided to drop the whole project and looked for another interest in
psychiatry. That is what led me to leave Perth for the far north of Western
Australia, to take the newly-created position as Regional Psychiatrist for the
Kimberley Health Region, based in the tiny town of Derby, WA (pop. 4600).

For six years, I travelled across that wild and beautiful part of the Great
State, working in near-total isolation to deliver psychiatric services to tiny
towns strung along the lonely Highway One and to remote Aboriginal
communities on the edges of the ancient deserts. I had no staff, no assistance
and, for the first few years, not even an office to call my own. There was
certainly nothing like a medical library, there was no internet and I remember
the day the first fax was installed. It was about as far from philosophy as
anybody could ever hope to go but it didn't work. Dealing with the Aboriginal
people, whose culture is probably less like Western culture than any on the
planet, forced me to examine the very notions of mental life, of mental
disorder and of culture. These, of course, are absolutely fundamental
questions in philosophy, and so I arrived back at the very questions I had
hoped to leave behind. Very often, travelling home at night, utterly alone on
the road, with the titanic thunderstorms of the northern monsoon towering
around me, I found myself tossing over ideas on the nature of belief, or of the
role of anxiety in causing depression in tribal peoples. I still had all my books,

of course, and often got home in the middle of the night and sat down to pore over one or other of the greats. And so the project wormed itself back into my life but, this time, I wasn't bothered when none of my friends or colleagues showed little interest.

When we left the Kimberley for Darwin, I had access to a library again but the pressures of work, of a young family and of building a house left little time for arcane questions of the nature of mental life. Several times, I put the matter away, then decided to have a final go at sorting out the questions. The result was a monograph called *The Future of Psychiatry* which, in short, didn't have a future. Thirty-two publishers rejected it so, in January, 2000, I put it on the Internet. There was a little interest around the world but nothing much. In September that year, the Olympic Games were held in Sydney and my children wanted to watch the opening ceremony on the television. Watching the hoopla, it seemed to me that people were more interested in kitsch than in the nature of mind. While people dressed as Vegemite jars waltzing with lawn-mowers projected Australia to the world, I promised myself that if there had been no interest in the project by the time of the next Games, in Athens, I would drop it entirely. Despite working on it, submitting papers, giving lectures at conferences and contacting publishers, August 2004 arrived and still there was no interest. Rather bitterly, I did as I had said and took up another project. I remember thinking how as a student years ago, while working alone on an isolated farm, I had found a copy of Charles Dickens' *David Copperfield*. This is said to be his most autobiographical work. One quote from his young hero always stuck in my mind: "I had no advice, no counsel, no encouragement, no consolation, no assistance, no support, of any kind, from anyone, that I can call to mind, as I hope to go to heaven!"

Finally, the silence had got too much. The author E.L. Doctorow asked: "After all, why compose fiction when you could be devoting your life to your appetites? Why wrestle with a book when you could be amassing a fortune? Why write when you could be shooting someone?" [1]. How much more difficult, then, to write a science for an establishment that doesn't want to hear of it.

However, the original work was still on the Internet and one day, a boutique publisher in the US contacted me with a publication proposal. That meant the whole work had to be rewritten to bring it up to date and to broaden it. *Humanizing Madness* was published by LH Press, of Ann Arbor, Michigan, in October 2007, just thirty-three years since I had first realized that Freud's idea of ego defenses could be better explained without invoking an unconscious. Slowly, the silence is giving way to curiosity and, *mirabile dictu*, interest and support. So on the strength of that support, I have completed the philosophical and practical sections of the project in this new book.

Beside the stated goals of this work, there are several themes that keep bobbing around. The first one is that modern psychiatry is deservedly headed for the scrap heap. The facts are blindingly obvious. Psychiatrists are losing control of their own field to psychologists, nurses, lawyers, social workers, accountants and administrators. Budgets are shrinking, facilities are closing, treatment is being rationed, patients are shoved out onto the streets. Within medicine, we are seen as rather silly people and medical students are voting with their feet by not taking up careers in this profession. The reason, as I have said so many times, is because we do not have a theory of mental disorder.

Unfortunately, most psychiatrists don't like being told this. In fact, it would be fair to say that the criticism provokes a hostile response from most parts of the profession. Oddly enough, it has never provoked any of those hostile people into saying: "Excuse me, but you're wrong. I have a copy of the standard scientific theory of mental disorder right here." They simply walk away, so I thought I should be a bit more forthright. In a letter to the then president of the Royal Australian and New Zealand College of Psychiatrists, I invited the College to participate in a public debate on the topic: "The RANZCP does not have a scientific model of mental disorder to guide its practice, teaching and research." The College declined on the basis that "...it is not a role of the College nor appropriate to debate publicly such issues." Granting the author of that letter, the current president of the College, all the respect he deserves, I think his letter is absolute rubbish. Examining the scientific basis of theories of mental disorder most definitely is part of the role of any professional psychiatric body. Pretending that it is not exposes my professional organization to accusations of a cover-up. Since the RANZCP has been told dozens of times that it doesn't have a scientific model of mental disorder, I cannot see how they imagine they might defend themselves against this most deadly of charges.

Similarly, the website of the American Psychiatric Association proclaims that it is "...the voice and conscience of modern psychiatry." There is no mention of a brain. The "mission" of its subsidiary body, the Institute on Psychiatric Services, is "...to train and support psychiatrists and other mental health professionals to provide quality care and leadership through the study of an array of clinical innovations and services necessary to meet the needs of individuals who suffer from mental illness, substance abuse, or other assaults to their mental health due to trauma or adverse social circumstances, in order to assure optimal care and hope of recovery." The model they use to teach psychiatrists how to intervene and what to avoid is nowhere in sight. Like all "mission statements" and "visions" and other window dressing, it is an exercise in vapid narcissism.

That illustrates the second theme, the stone-walling refusal of orthodox psychiatry to examine and criticize what they do. If and when the general public realizes that this is the case, I expect that the decline or our profession will accelerate very sharply. I am utterly unable to understand why any psychiatrist should believe that the taxpayers and insurers will want to continue paying for a service with no rational basis. President Obama's Council of Economic Advisers reports that, in the US today, health care consumes some 18% of GDP. By 2040, when my children will still be in their forties, it is expected that health will consume over one third of GDP [2]. That's 34c in every dollar earned or produced in that country, and mental health care will be a large and growing part of that sum. I would like a member of the psychiatric establishment to explain to me (and to the taxpayers) why a profession that has no rational scientific basis should be allowed to get its hands on such a large chunk of the GDP. One day in the not-too-distant future, people are going to wake up to the fact that they are being gulled. And that will be the end of psychiatry as we know it. Unfortunately, if psychiatry finally dies of inanity, what will take its place will be worse. How can I be so sure? Because the natural progression of ideas is that a new and better idea forces the old concepts aside but, outside psychiatry, there is nothing. Nobody has any better ideas. Nothing can come from nothing.

However, and this is my main theme, all this could all change. The biocognitive model outlined in these two books provides a framework for a formal, rational model of mental disorder and how to intervene to correct it. That should be cause for celebration in psychiatric circles: at last, a model of madness. Better still, it is a model for psychiatry: of all the professions with an interest in mental disorder, only a medical practitioner can understand it. A psychiatrist using this model can work alone: I should know, as I developed it when I was the world's most isolated psychiatrist. Better still, the model allows dramatic reductions in the costs of mental health care. It reduces the burden of mental disorder, by keeping people out of hospitals, getting them back home and back to work much earlier, with huge reductions in the costs of medication, investigations, support and ancillary services, etc. This model will lead to the next big wave of closures of mental hospitals. However, that does not mean we can allow a repetition of the last wave, when the patients were simply drugged to the eyeballs and pushed out into the streets, into dosshouses and into prison.

Armed with the biocognitive model, psychiatrists can say to governments: We can cut costs and give people a vastly improved quality of life. I think any government would be keen to hear that. Any patient would be more than pleased to hear it, too. That way, we could recover some of our prestige and start to attract bright young doctors into the profession by showing them something very, very exciting, future for psychiatry.

The reasonable man adapts himself to the world.
The unreasonable man persists in trying to adapt the world to himself.
All progress, therefore, depends on the unreasonable man.
GB Shaw: *The Revolutionist's Handbook*

References

Chapter 1: Defining Limits to Biological Reductionism

1. Carr G. Who do you think you are? A survey of the brain. *The Economist* Supplement, December 23rd 2006. Available online at www.economist.com/surveys.

2. Kandel ER. *Psychiatry, psychoanalysis and the new biology of mind.* Washington, DC: American Psychiatric Publishing. 2005.

3. El-Hai J. *The lobotomist: A maverick medical genius and his tragic quest to rid the world of mental illne*ss. New York: Wiley, 2007. ISBN 978-0470098301.

4. Jansson B. Controversial neurosurgery resulted in a Nobel Prize (Oct. 1998). Available at www.Nobelprize.org, Nobel Prizes in Medicine. Accessed July 23rd 2007.

5. Kandel ER. *In search of memory: the emergence of a new science of mind.* New York: Norton, 2006.

6. Kandel ER, Schwartz JH, Jessell TM. *Principles of neuroscience.* 4th Edn. New York: McGraw Hill, 2000.

7. Kandel ER, Schwartz JH, Jessell TM. *Essentials of neural science and behavior.* Norwalk, Conn: Appleton Lange, 1995 (new edition is planned).

8. Masson JM. *The assault on truth: Freud's suppression of the seduction theory.* New York: Simon and Schuster, 1998.

9. Crews F (Ed.). *Unauthorized Freud: Doubters confront a legend.* New York: Penguin Putnam, 1998.

10. McLaren N. *Humanizing madness: psychiatry and the cognitive neurosciences.* Ann Arbor, MI: Future Psychiatry Press, 2007. ISBN 978-1-932690-39-2

11. Dancy J, Sosa E. *A companion to epistemology.* Malden, MA: Blackwell, 1992. ISBN 978-0-631-19258-9.

Chapter 2: Turing Computability and the Brain: Critical Implications for Biological Psychiatry

1. McLaren N. *Humanizing madness: Psychiatry and the cognitive neurosciences.* 2007. Ann Arbor, MI.: Future Psychiatry Press.

2. McLaren N. Kandel's 'New Science of Mind' for Psychiatry and the limits to biological reductionism: a critical review. *Ethical human psychology and psychiatry* 2008; 10: 109-121. Expanded version at Ch. 1.

3. Kandel ER. *Psychiatry, psychoanalysis and the new biology of mind.* 2005. Washington: APA Publishing.

4. Turing AM. On computable numbers, with an application to the Entscheidungs problem. *Proceedings of the london mathematical society* (1936 - 37) Series 2; 42:230-65. Available online: See Wikipedia.

5. Turing AM. Computing machinery and intelligence. *Mind* 1950; 59: 433-60.

6. Crews F. *Unauthorised Freud: doubters confront a legend.* Penguin Putnam; New York; 1998.

7. McKenzie BD. *Behaviourism and the limits of scientific method.* Routledge and Kegan Paul: London; 1977.

Chapter 3: Science and the Psychiatric Publishing Industry

Dean ET. *Shook over hell: Post-traumatic stress, vietnam and the civil war.* 1997; Harvard University Press: Cambridge, Mass.

1. McLaren N. *Humanizing madness: Psychiatry and the cognitive neurosciences.* 2007; Ann Arbor, Mi.: Future Psychiatry Press. .

2. McLaren N. Kandel's 'New Science of Mind' for Psychiatry and the limits to biological reductionism: a critical review. *Ethical human psychology and psychiatry* 2008; 10: 109-121.

3. Lakatos I, Musgrave A (Eds). *Criticism and the growth of knowledge.* Cambridge: University Press, 1970.

4. Kuhn TS. *The structure of scientific revolutions.* 2nd Edition, 1970. Chicago, Ill: University Press (International Encyclopedia of Unified Science, Vol. 2, No. 2)

5. Young SN. The neurobiology of human social behavior: an important but neglected topic. *J Psychiat. Neurosci.* 2008; 233(5): 391-2.

6. McLaren N. Interactive dualism as a partial solution to the mind-brain problem for psychiatry. *Medical Hypotheses* 2006; 66: 1165-1173.

7. Bennett MR. Development of the concept of the mind. *Aust NZ J Psychiat* 2007; 41:943-956.

8. Bennett MR. Dual constraints on synapse formation and regression in schizophrenia... *Aust N Z J Psychiat* 2008; 42:662-677.

9. Popper KR. *Conjectures and refutations: the growth of scientific knowledge.* London: Routledge, 1972.

10. Popper KR. *Objective knowledge: an evolutionary approach.* Oxford: Clarendon Press, 1972.

11. Stevenson L. *Seven theories of human nature.* Oxford: University Press, 1974.

12. Ioannidis JPA (2005) Why Most Published Research Findings Are False. *PLoS Med* 2(8): e124 doi:10.1371/journal.pmed.0020124. Cited November 8th 2008.

13. Young NS, Ioannidis JPA, Al-Ubaydli O (2008) Why Current Publication Practices May Distort Science. *PLoS Med* 5(10): e201 doi:10.1371/ journal.pmed. 0050201. Cited November 8th 2008.

14. Engel GL. The need for a new medical model: a challenge for biomedicine. *Science* 1977; 196:129-136.

Chapter 4: The Case for a Mentalist Psychiatry

1. Luria AR. *Higher cortical functions in man.* New York: Basic Books, 1977.

2. Dennett DC. *Consciousness explained.* London: Penguin Books, 1993

3. Peters RS. *The concept of motivation.* London: Routledge & Kegan Paul, 1960.

4. Dennett DC. *Brainstorms: philosophical essays on mind and psychology.* Hassocks, Sussex: Harvester Press, 1978.

5. Dennett DC. *The intentional stance.* Cambridge, Mass: Bradford Books/MIT Press, 1989.

6. MacKenzie BD. *Behaviorism and the limits of scientific method.* London: Routledge & Kegan Paul, 1977.

7. Skinner BF. Behaviorism at fifty. In: Wann TW. *Behaviorism and phenomenology.* Chicago: University Press, 1964

8. Skinner BF. *Beyond Freedom and Dignity.* New York: Bantam Books, 1972.

9. Skinner BF. *About behaviorism.* New York: Random House, 1974.

10. Skinner BF. Why I am not a cognitive psychologist. In: *Reflections on behaviorism and society.* New York: Knopf, 1974.

11. Tolman EC. "A Behaviorist theory of ideas." *Psychol. Rev.* 33:352-369, 1926.

12. Engel GL. The care of the patient: art or science? *Johns hopkins medical journal* 1977; 140:222-232.

Chapter 5. Toward A Molecular Resolution of the Mind-Body Problem for Psychiatry

1. McLaren N. *Humanizing madness: psychiatry and the cognitive neurosciences* 2007. Ann Arbor, Mi.: Future Psychiatry Press. .

2. Chalmers DJ. *The conscious mind: in search of a fundamental theory.* Oxford: University Press, 1996.

3. Dennett DC. *Consciousness explained.* London: Penguin Books, 1993.

4. Popper KR, Eccles JC. *The self and its brain.* London: Springer, 1981.

5. Turing AM. On computable numbers, with an application to the Entscheidungsproblem. *Proceedings of the london mathematical society* (1936 - 37) Series 2; 42:230-65. Available on line: See author entry in Wikipedia.

6. Turing AM. Computing machinery and intelligence. *Mind* 1950; 59: 433-60.

7. Mountcastle VB. The columnar organization of the neocortex. *Brain* 1997; 120: 701-722.

8. Bressler SL, Tognoli E. Operational principles of neurocognitive networks. *International journal of psychophysiology* 2006; 60: 139–148

9. Sompayrac L. *How the immune system works.* 3rd Edn. Malden, Mass.: Blackwell, 2008.

Chapter 6: Embodied Logic

1. Kriegeskorte N, Mur M, Ruff DA, Kiani R, Bodurka J, Esteky H, Tanaka K, Bandettini PA. Matching categorical object representations in inferior temporal cortex of man and monkey. *Neuron* 2008; 60: 126-1141. Available on line.

2. Logic Gates. Wikipedia. Accessed 31.12.08. (this article gives diagrams demonstrating each type of gate). See also: Boolean Algebra.

3. Kandel ER. *Psychiatry, psychoanalysis and the new biology of mind.* Washington, DC: American Psychiatric Publishing. 2005.

4. Kandel ER, Jessel TM, Schwartz JH. *Principles of neuroscience.* New York: McGraw Hill, 2000.

5. Pocock G, Richards CD. *Human physiology: the basis of medicine.*

6. Purves D. *Neuroscience.* 4th Edn. Sunderland, Conn: Sinauer Assoc., 2007. ISBN 978-0878936977.

7. Hubel DH, Wiesel TN. *Brain and visual perception.* New York: Oxford University Press, 2005.

8. Benjamin PR, Kemenes G, Kemenes I. Non-synaptic neuronal mechanisms of learning and memory in gastropod molluscs. *Frontiers in bioscience* 2008; 113: 4051-57.

9. McLaren N. *Humanizing madness: psychiatry and the cognitive neurosciences* 2007. Ann Arbor, Mi.: Future Psychiatry Press. ISBN 9781932690392.

10. Turing AM. Computing machinery and intelligence. *Mind* 1950; 59: 433-60.

11. Hameroff S. Quantum consciousness: the new frontier in brain science. Available at www.quantumconsciousness.org. Accessed Dec. 30th 2008.

12. Bressler SL, Tognoli E. Operational principles of neurocognitive networks. *International Journal of Psychophysiology* 2006; 60: 139–148

13. Hebb DO. *The organization of behavior: a neuropsychological theory.* New York: Wiley, 1957.

14. Zhang W, Linden DJ. The other side of the engram: experience-driven changes in neuronal excitability. *Nature Reviews Neuroscience.* 2003; 4: 885-900.

15. Carew CJ, Sahley CL. Invertebrate learning and memory: from behavior to molecules. *Annual Review of Neuroscience.* 1986; 9: 435-487.

16. Fulton D, Kemenes I, Andrews RJ, Benjamin PR. Time-window for cooling distinguishes the effects of hypothermia and protein synthesis inhibition on the consolidation of long-term memory. *Neurobiology of Learning and Memory* 2008; 90: 651-654.

17. Benjamin PR, Kemenes G, Kemenes I. Non-synaptic neuronal mechanisms of learning and memory in gastropod molluscs. *Frontiers in Bioscience* 13, 4051-4057, May 1, 2008.

18. Jones NG, Kemenes G, Kemenes I, Benjamin PR. A persistent cellular change in a single modulatory neuron contributes to associative long term memory. *Current biology* 13: 1064-9, 2003.

19. Somgyi P, Tamas G, Lujan R, Buhl EH. Salient features of synaptic organization in the cortex. *Brain research reviews* 1998; 26:113-135 (this excellent paper shows much more detailed diagrams of sub-modular "cortical wiring").

Chapter 7: The Biocognitive Model

1. Kandel ER. *Psychiatry, psychoanalysis and the new biology of mind.* Washington, DC: American Psychiatric Publishing. 2005.

2. McLaren N. *Humanizing madness: psychiatry and the cognitive neurosciences* 2007. Ann Arbor, Mi.: Future Psychiatry Press. .

3. Chalmers DJ. *The conscious mind: In search of a fundamental theory.* Oxford: University Press, 1996.

4. Ruse M. Taking darwin seriously: A naturalistic approach to philosophy. Amherst, NY: Prometheus Books, 1998.

5. Luria AR. *Higher cortical functions in man.* New York: Basic Books, 1980.

6. Chomsky N. *New horizons in the study of language and mind.* Cambridge: University Press, 2000.

7. Seligman MEP. Phobias and preparedness. *Behavior therapy* 1971; 2: 307-21.

8. Oehman A, Mineka S. The malicious serpent: snakes as a prototypical stimulus for an evolved module of fear. *Current directions in psychological science* 2003; 12: 5-9.

9. Pocock G, Richards CD. *Human physiology: The basis of medicine.* 3rd Ed. Oxford: University Press, 2006.

10. Stevenson L, Haberman DL. *Ten theories of human nature.* New York: Oxford University Press, 2009.

Chapter 8: Language as a Test of the Biocognitive Model

1. McLaren N. *Humanizing madness: Psychiatry and the cognitive neurosciences* 2007. Ann Arbor, Mi.: Future Psychiatry Press. .

2. Lycan WG. *Philosophy of language: a contemporary introduction.* 2nd Edn. New York: Routledge, 2008.

3. Chomsky N. *New horizons in the study of language and mind.* New York: Cambridge University Press, 2000.

4. Luria AR. *Higher cortical functions in man.* New York: Basic Books, 1980.

5. Popper KR, Eccles JC. *The self and its brain.* London: Springer, 1981.

6. Van Lawick Goodall J. *In the shadow of man.* Fontana: London, 1974.

7. Williams M. *Problems of Knowledge: a critical introduction to epistemology.* New York: Oxford University Press, 2001.

8. Dancy J, Sosa E (Eds). *A companion to epistemology.* Malden, MA: Blackwell, 1993.

9. Engel GL. The biopsychosocial model and the education of health professionals. *Annals of the new york academy of sciences* 1978; 310: 169-181.

Chapter 9: The Biocognitive Model and Human Nature

1. Meggitt MJ. *Desert People: a study of the Walpiri Aborigines of Central Australia.* Sydney: Angus and Robertson, 1962.

2. Berndt RM, Berndt CH. *The world of the first Australians: Aboriginal traditional life, past and present.* Sydney: Rigby, 1985.

3. Spindler K. *The man in the ice: the story of a Neolithic man frozen in a glacier for 5000 years.* London: Weidenfeld and Nicholson, 1993 (Eng. Translation 1994).

4. Brown DE. *Human universals.* New York: McGraw Hill, 1991.

Chapter 10: Personality

1. Kandel ER. *Psychiatry, psychoanalysis and the new biology of mind.* Washington, DC: American Psychiatric Publishing. 2005.

2. Kandel ER. *In search of memory: the emergence of a new science of mind.* New York: Norton, 2006.

3. *The Economist* Dec. 22nd 2007, p118:

4. Stekel W, quoted in Brown JAC. *Freud and the Post-Freudians.* London: Penguin, 1964.

5. Horwitz AV, Wakefield JC. *The Loss of sadness: how psychiatry transformed normal sorrow into depressive disorder.* New York: Oxford University Press, 2007.

6. Perini S, Titov N, Andrews G. Clinician-assisted internet-based treatment is effective for depression: Randomized controlled trial. *Australian and New Zealand Journal of Psychiatry* 2009; 43:571-578.

Chapter 11: *Circus Vitiosus*

1. Watson JB. *Behaviorism.* New York: Norton, 1925.

2. Skinner BF. *Beyond Freedom and Dignity.* New York: Knopf, 1971.

3. Sompayrac L. *How the immune system works.* 3rd Ed. Malden, Mass.: Blackwell, 2008.

4. Pocock G, Richards CD. *Human Physiology: The basis of medicine.* 3rd Ed. Oxford: University Press, 2006.

5. Perini S, Titov N, Andrews G. Clinician-assisted Internet-based treatment is effective for depression: Randomized controlled trial. *Australian and New Zealand Journal of Psychiatry* 2009; 43:571-578.

6. Stevenson L, Haberman DL. *Ten Theories of Human Nature.* 5th Edn. New York: Oxford University Press, 2009.

Chapter 12: The Culture of Complacency

1. Dean ET. Shook over hell: Post-traumatic stress, Vietnam and the Civil War. Harvard: University Press, 1997.

2. Broad Wm, Wade N. *Betrayers of the truth: fraud and deceit in the halls of science.* London: Century, 1983.

3. McLaren N. Science and the psychiatric publishing industry. *Ethical Human Psychology and Psychiatry.* 2009; 11:29-36.

4. Bloch S. A call to authors: three solid reasons to publish in the *ANZJP. Australian and New Zealand Journal of Psychiatry* 2002: 36; 1-3.

Epilogue

1. Doctorow EL. *Creationists. Selected essays 1993-2006.* New York: Random House, 2006.

2. *The Economist* (Asian Edition). June 6-12, 2009, p34.

Index

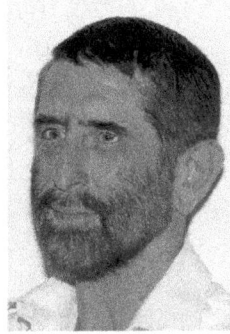